CROHN'S AND COLITIS FIX

Advance Praise

Inna is a passionate healer that has revealed her personal journey to heal her own IBD. Through her journey Inna explains how she was able to improve her body's ability to heal itself, though very simple and specific diet modifications, tests and unique treatments and supplements. Essentially, this can become your IBD how-to-heal support guide! Surely, this is a must read for anyone looking for options on their IBD healing journey."

—**Jeffrey A. Morrison, M.D.**, CNS

Crohn's and Colitis Fix is an essential book for anyone with IBDs who wants to feel better and understand the complexity of the illness. Dr. Inna Lukyanovsky has created a clear 10-week program that incorporates her knowledge as a Doctor of Pharmacy, experience of a Crohn's patient in full remission and an expertise in Functional Medicine. Dr. Inna presents such a comprehensive, complementary style medicine guide to IBDs which involves so much more than the traditional approach.

—**Mark Hyman, MD**, Ten-time #1 New York Times bestselling author, Director, Cleveland Clinic Center for Functional Medicine, Founder and Director, The UltraWellness Center

Dr. Inna Lukyanovsky is such important asset in getting great gut health. Smart gut microbiome support is a staple for thyroid warriors as much as thyroid support is often necessary for patients with inflammatory bowels. Both autoimmune conditions have many things in common and Hashimoto's protocol is also very involved with lifestyle interventions. This book will surely be a classic for lifestyle changes in Crohn's and colitis.

—**Izabella Wentz**, PharmD, Author *Hashimoto's Thyroiditis: Lifestyle Interventions for Finding and Treating the Root Cause and Hashimoto's Protocol: A 90-Day Plan for Reversing Thyroid Symptoms and Getting Your Life Back*. www.thyroidpharmacist.com

CROHN'S AND COLITIS FIX

10 WEEK PLAN

for Reversing IBD Symptoms and Getting Rid of Fatigue

INNA LUKYANOVSKY, PharmD

NEW YORK

LONDON • NASHVILLE • MELBOURNE • VANCOUVER

CROHN'S AND COLITIS FIX
10 WEEK PLAN *for Reversing IBD Symptoms and Getting Rid of Fatigue*

Published in New York, New York, by Morgan James Publishing in partnership with Difference Press. Morgan James is a trademark of Morgan James, LLC. www.MorganJamesPublishing.com

ISBN 978-1-64279-226-3 paperback
ISBN 978-1-64279-227-0 eBook
Library of Congress Control Number: 2018909836

Cover Design by:
Rachel Lopez
www.r2cdesign.com

Interior Design by:
Bonnie Bushman
The Whole Caboodle Graphic Design

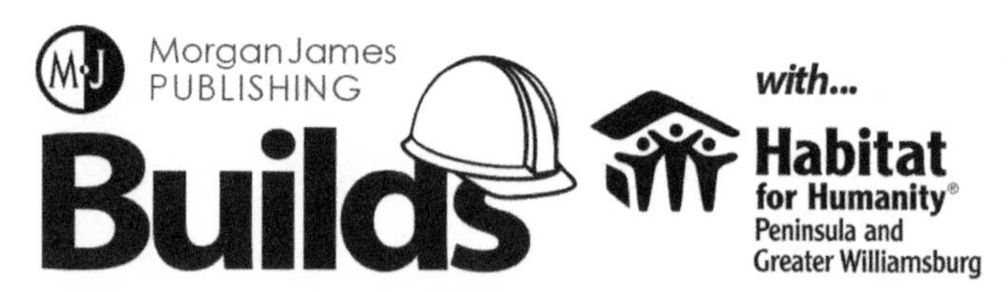

DEDICATION

For Ethan, Ashton, and Sam who always believe in Mom's "magical" abilities to heal. May you always live with integrity, love for learning, and never-ending enthusiasm.

TABLE OF CONTENTS

FOREWORD

Crohn's and Colitis Fix by my good friend and colleague of many years, Inna Lukyanovsky, is an excellent resource for people suffering with digestive disorders who want to better understand the underlying causes of chronic GI problems. Her work in this area for the past many years has culminated in this ten-week program that provides clear guidelines for assessment and treatment options using a functional medicine approach to all-too-common digestive problems suffered by millions of people worldwide.

As my twenty-five years of practice have unfolded I have seen more and more severe cases of Crohn's and colitis coming into the clinic, with people suffering from ever more extreme food reactions and food allergies, gluten-related problems, and the like. We are clearly becoming sicker and more stressed and the elusive goal of optimum health seems out of range to many people. I believe Dr. Inna Lukyanovsky's book creates an opening, an opportunity for people who have been all but given up on by conventional medicine to begin to piece back together their health puzzle and restore their basic body systems to a healthy status, using hormone balancing, GI improvements, and learning how nutrients and detoxification play an integrated role in recovery from chronic illnesses.

Please do yourself a favor and dive into this book and begin to unravel your specific health concerns using a functional medicine approach.

Yours in Health,

Daniel Kalish, Founder of Kalish Wellness, Functional Medicine Pioneer, Founder of Kalish Institute and Author of *The Kalish Method: Healing the Body, Mapping the Mind.*

INTRODUCTION

"Health is like money, we never have
a true idea of its value until we lose it."
—Josh Billings

What's Going on with My Body? I'm Too Busy to Be Sick.

Julie had been a happy, cheerful, and optimistic person since she was a little girl. She was always very intuitive and noticed, as a child, that the way she behaved was annoying to her friends. It drove them crazy to see how happy she could act. She would start skipping when she saw the blue skies or when someone took her out on a trip. Little things made her excited. And yes, she grew up, but she remained that positive little girl inside.

What is happening to me? I'm so exhausted, these terrible fevers, these horrible, bloody runs. I have an infant and a toddler. I need to take care of them. I must figure this out, thought Julie. *There's no reason I should be feeling this way.* Julie was concerned and questioned why she was not healing. The doctors in the ICU were diagnosing her with everything possible, like pneumonia, sepsis, or other infections, but they were never sure. And then, finally, a diagnosis—ulcerative colitis—came as a shock.

The medications were taken, but Julie wasn't improving much. There were so many antibiotics that Julie thought her gut must be sterile now—no bug could be living in there anymore! And the symptoms just continued. She was so exhausted that she would fall asleep quickly, but she would often wake up at night from the pain or from having to go to the bathroom. The physical abdominal pain was often so bad that it would wake her up at night, almost like a nightmare. Once she was up at night, the thoughts would run wild and the fear of dying would creep in, and the fear of not being able to spend time with the kids, and the fear of not being able to pay the mortgage, and the fear of not being able to work because she always needed "to go." *This can't continue,* she thought. *I need a break.*

On the following trip to the doctor's office she complained that she had trouble sleeping and that she was very depressed. You would think that would be expected, that the person who was in pain, constantly embarrassed about having diarrhea, bloating, gas, and the other wonderful stuff that came along with this illness, would be likely to start feeling this way. So, the next recommendation from her physician was to see a psychiatrist. She was seen by the psychiatrist for a very short appointment and left the office with anti-depressant and anti-anxiety prescriptions. She came home and finally felt really depressed. She couldn't understand why she was given medications by a psychiatrist when she was not a psychiatric patient—or why she had even agreed to go there.

Then the next stage came. Julie didn't want to do anything. She didn't feel like eating, drinking, or taking her medications. Being super sensitive and even intuitive, Julie felt that her husband was growing tired of this new situation. She was just waiting for him to come in one day and tell her it was over. And maybe, just maybe, she didn't need to wait until he said it; maybe it was time to say it herself. But, what about the kids? How would they handle a single mom situation?

So, with her focus on getting healthy or else, Julie wrote herself a letter that was meant for future-Julie in ten years. This is what she wrote to herself:

Dear Julie,

I know that you've been through a lot, but you came out of it stronger and healthier than you've ever been. Look how much you've accomplished in ten years. You are now a medical doctor, seeing patients, helping them heal, and traveling a lot for work to learn new methods. You are a mom of two wonderful kids and your husband is so supportive. Your house is incredible, impeccable, just a dream come true home with a beautiful princess staircase, modern kitchen, and super cozy bedrooms. I believed in you and I always knew you would be the healthiest, happiest, and most gorgeous forty-year-old gal.

Your journey made you stronger and wiser and I'm thrilled that you are me in ten years. Thank you for taking all the steps to heal. Thank you for sticking with a program and believing in yourself and your healing. Thank you for showing me the way and most of all, thank you for not giving up!

Sincerely yours,
YOU ten years younger
P.S I hope you get this letter on your 40th birthday and that your next ten years will be as amazing or even more amazing than this decade.

Julie printed the letter and sealed it. She placed the letter where she kept her most important documents and letters, smiled, and went to sleep.

The next morning her first thought was about her appearance. Julie thought that if she wanted to physically feel a certain way, she should look a certain way too. She wanted to appear light, lean, and healthy looking. She pictured herself sitting elegantly, eating dinner with her back straight, with her fork in her left hand and her knife in the right one. She was almost daydreaming, imagining herself looking healthy. Julie went downstairs, got her computer, and searched for "natural solutions for IBDs."

Her road to healing was somewhat bumpy, yet she always remained focused on her goal. And her goal was complete healing. With the help of naturopathic and functional solutions, her willingness to stick with the healing program, and her positive energy, she was able to get back on track, and now she's in full health. This book will help you do the same.

This book is about healing your digestive mess. We often talk about treatment plans, we often discuss the problems and illnesses of others, and we often feel empathetic for those who are sick, but this book is about actually setting your intentions to heal Crohn's, colitis or other digestive illness and keep on going toward your goal. In this book, you will find practical steps to improve your chronic digestive disease. You will also find the tools and the functional medicine methods for gut healing.

If you are looking for a book that is the next magic pill or a plan to heal without doing anything at all, this isn't that type of book. The healing process is very complex, and functional medicine looks at all aspects of human health as a complex system, including emotions, stress, environment, toxins, microbiome, and more.

Crohn's disease and ulcerative colitis affect millions of people. This number is growing, but so is the research for Crohn's and colitis alternative, nutraceutical, and complementary treatments.

This book is about waking you up and helping you reset and restore your gastrointestinal flora. It will help you balance your gut microbiome, and it will help you figure out more about the importance of immune system response for your gut healing. It will teach you how toxins play a role in your illness. This book can help you become more proactive and be in better control of your health. It can teach you how to get more energy and how to balance your mind and gut better.

This book is a great tool for those that believe their digestive health is super important to them. It will be a tremendous benefit to those that are digging and looking not to just patch up their symptoms, but, instead to actually heal their root cause.

Here, I will share my journey with Crohn's disease and how I got to full remission. Health is important. Gut health is responsible for many other human body functions and systems including our brain, skeletal, muscular, and immune systems. If you recognize the importance of a healthy gut and a healthy immune system, you know that you would work at making it better. Healing your gut, sharing with others, empowering other patients, and empowering your children to eat better—you are on your journey to heal your beautiful tummy and the tummies of your loved ones.

If you've been through the merry-go-round of numerous doctor visits, hours of waiting, x-ray series, barium, MRIs with contrast, surgeries, and other "fun" stuff you go through when you have a chronic digestive disease, you know that you are willing to do anything to feel better. You spent hours doing acupuncture, acupressure, and massage therapies and you feel better but not great? And you tried yoga, suction cup therapies, bioenergy, and meditation and you feel better but not where you want to be? Maybe you are even sitting there thinking about trying fecal transplant or parasite ingestion because you read on some blog that it worked for Crohn's patients. I'd like you to take a breath and think about your healing. There's another way that works. It worked for me.

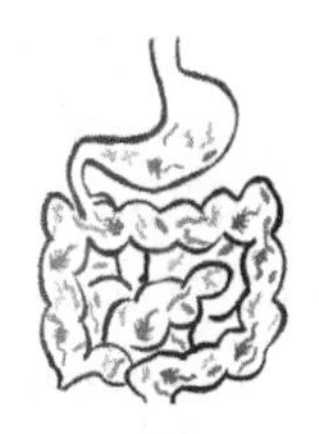

Chapter 1
MY JOURNEY

"Although the world is full of suffering,
it is also full of the overcoming of it."
—Helen Keller

Journey with Crohn's Disease

I knew that I would be a health care professional since I was a little girl. I loved my toy doctor's kit. I loved taking care of my family. I loved how assured the doctor always seemed. I even loved the trips to the pharmacy when I had to go with my grandma. Where I grew up, the pharmacies looked very different. They were old fashioned with glass counters, pharmacists and other personnel were dressed all in white, and oh, that smell of eucalyptus oil, it was intoxicating. I stared at the counter, looking at the glass rods used for mixing creams and couldn't wait to come home to use them to heal my dolls. I even made my grandma buy me first aid supplies that were completely useless to her so that I could enjoy my playtime.

I also chose my profession because I couldn't watch my grandma suffer. She was always having stomach problems and lost a large chunk of her large intestine due to chronic inflammation. At that time they didn't call it Crohn's or colitis, but that's what it probably was. So, I wanted to make a difference for her, to create the magic pill in the future so her stomach would stop hurting. Little did I know that I would get a Crohn's diagnosis myself. Well, maybe the universe had this plan for me.

The reason I wrote this book was because it was a natural next thing for me to do. I accomplished a lot as a health care professional, and I've dealt with so much as a Crohn's patient, that it just became an absolute next thing for me to do.

I've always procrastinated to write the book that I had wanted to write for so long, I've always procrastinated. I planned and I hoped and I planned again to eventually come up with the book for Crohn's that wouldn't just be a next book for IBD (Inflammatory Bowel Disease), but a book that was a "know how" to leave the symptoms behind A book on how to fix the gut more effectively without the fear, without "the what if it doesn't work," "what if it's just another self-help book that claims to help IBD patients." I wanted to write a very different book for a *real* Crohn's or colitis patient where it's easy to follow the steps, where it's easy to fit the suggestions into your lifestyle, and it can work as well as it did for me.

In the beginning of my healing journey, I was in a place of fear, pain, and despair, with lots of questions and lots of moments where I felt numb, almost paralyzed. I thought, *Is this it? Is this how it's going to feel for the rest of my life? Is this how I'm going to spend my holidays? Is this how I am going to take care of my kids? Is this how I am going to work?* I was lucky, somehow my husband made me believe that I was going to be okay—and that's super important to believe in your healing. One morning, during one of my flares, he told me that we would absolutely find something that would work. He looked at me with such certainty, and he's such a kind and honest man. At that moment I had no doubt. That feeling of real hope carried me through the rough days and nights, and that belief made me strong enough to get to the next step of my journey, the step where I asked myself, *What am I going to try now? I've tried the traditional route without much help. I've already lost my hope once, I'm not going to lose hope again.* My husband was right; I would find something that would work.

What happened in my case? After I had my first child I had mild colitis symptoms and was misdiagnosed with ulcerative colitis. I thought that was bad and I was scared. Unfortunately, this kind of misdiagnosis still happens when ulcerative colitis presents as Crohn's and vice versa, especially with mild symptoms. The symptoms started going away slowly with medicine, and I thought my colitis was gone.

When I was delivering my second child it all came back with a vengeance. The diagnosis was now Crohn's disease and the symptoms were so severe that I felt completely debilitated. I went through a nightmare that no one should ever live through. I thought to myself, *How did this happen? What did I do to deserve this suffering?*

By the way, I never ask those types of questions anymore. It's not healthy for the soul to dwell on "Why's" and "What's." Let it go. Start fresh. You must think positive no matter what.

There were numerous points during my illness when I said to myself, *No more. I must try taking more control over my health and get myself better. I am a healthcare professional, after all.* But it did take time and different circumstances to start climbing out of that negative state.

When I was prescribed medications, it was very difficult to take them, since I'm a pharmacist and I was keenly aware of all of the side effects of the drugs that I had to take. Every time I took a pill I thought of the mechanism of action or pharmacology of that drug and all of the horrible side effects that accompanied it; and I experienced many of them. My mood was terrible on Prednisone. My white blood count was ridiculous on Remicade and 6-MP. I started reading all I could about IBDs.

While I was lying in bed after an ICU visit I started writing a book on my positive aspects, and that kept my spirits and hopes up. My babysitter at that time was using a unique, old Eastern method of healing and gave me a book which included instructions on meditation, as well as certain physical exercises that I thought were too hard to do at that time. She insisted that I get out of bed and try those exercises. I wish I had stuck with that program then. It would probably have sped up my healing journey. But then I wouldn't have found and fallen in love with functional medicine.

My complementary treatments journey started. I went to try acupuncture, and the doctor practicing it was trained in Asia. He even had those very thick needles that they don't use anymore. It was painful, and I was happy—yes, happy. I thought through the pain I would heal faster and I would feel better sooner. The treatments did improve my digestion. I tried some other herbs later and some homeopathic medications that slowly decreased the inflammation. I also found a medical doctor that practiced non-traditional holistic medicine, who made a big difference for me with more appropriate dietary changes, some IV infusions, and chelation treatments.

Since I did get some positive results from the acupuncture doctor, I thought I would try some of his Chinese herbs, too. That didn't agree with me much. I was feeling a shift, though, so I was already getting excited about my next steps in the healing journey and thinking of what those steps could be.

The next thing I tried was unorthodox. My sister-in-law called me on the same day that I heard about John of God. My sister-in-law told me that she and her daughter were going to see John of God and that she would love for me to join them. I immediately said yes. John of God's Casa is a world-known spiritual healing center located in a secluded, almost hidden, area of Brazil. John of God himself is a medium who accepts a few spirits, depending on the day or the hour, to advise the visitors who are seeking healing of the mind and body. Not everyone is a believer, but I was certainly ready for a miracle then. This was a trip I won't forget, the cold summer (which meant winter in Brazil), the invisible and visible surgeries, the peaceful time healing, that meditation room, the freezing healing waterfalls, and the crystal room that felt like it was heating me up from the inside; it was all surreal. I did get a fever there, too. Although fevers didn't surprise me much—I had those fevers for a while now—they did feel somewhat different in the Casa, as if this fever would finally break the illness.

My mother came on that trip with me and it was a bigger life changer for her than me. She was a complete skeptic before. She didn't believe in anything that didn't make sense, and John of God certainly didn't make sense to her. But that was before she saw him operate on someone's eye with a knife without anesthesia, and without much blood. I don't know why I was not chosen to go through the line that saw this, but I guess it was because I was a believer before I even came, so I didn't need validation. The time came to return home, and while I wasn't sure that the trip had made any physical difference for me, I was convinced this trip had a meaning. Now I know that it did. I came back knowing that I would find the way for sure and I would even help others to heal.

Coming back from Brazil was exciting. I felt like a celebrity since everyone was calling to ask me how it went. I had many people with cancer diagnoses calling me for trip suggestions, and I was thrilled to share. It was time to get back into my life, and while at that time my number of bathroom trips decreased, they still ruled my life. I still couldn't go out for too long without looking for a bathroom. And, as I previously mentioned, the medications didn't work, but now they made me *so* fatigued. I told my doctor that I was getting off of the medications. I took a risk, a big risk, and I tapered off the medications and eventually discontinued them while starting my first round of nutraceuticals. It was super scary. *What if I get worse, just like the doctor said? What if I have to go to the hospital again? I have small kids, I'm so scared.* And although I absolutely do not recommend stopping medications on your own, ever, it was my personal choice. I took a huge risk. I could have gotten worse, but I didn't. And I stopped having that fatigue.

The next person who made a difference for me was a holistic clinical nutritionist from California who was visiting my friend's mother, and she thought he could help. I didn't even know that there could be such a thing as a holistic nutritionist! I was listening to him, taking notes, copying his every word. I took a trip to the nearest health food store and spent a fortune there. This was 2003. And, you guessed it, the food from the health food store in 2003 was not tasty at all. I didn't care! I believed it would help and I had to do what I had to do. And you know what? Now, when I hear a client say that they don't want to try this or that, because it is not sweet and delicious enough, I ask if they really want to get rid of their problem.

The next important figure in my journey was Jordan Rubin and his book *Patient Heal Thyself. It was* about how he healed his Crohn's. I purchased his probiotics, and that's when my love affair with probiotics started. On my next visit to my gastro I mentioned taking probiotics and I got a huge laugh from him. "If probiotics worked, then everyone would be taking them! If you show me research that proves that probiotics work, I would be more understanding," he said. Well, that gave me a mission for my probiotic and gut microbiome research that will be never-ending learning. I recently finished my doctorate in pharmacy and the topic of my paper was the clinical effectiveness of probiotics in Crohn's and colitis. Probiotics are not made the same. There is so much room for continuous research, both on the microbiology and genetics ends. Probiotics work. It's a whole new science on its own. And I love my science!

Another thing I did that I'm happy about was mercury amalgam (silver filling) removal. Although still controversial, the amalgam removal is often recommended by naturopathic, holistic, and integrative practitioners because of the association with systemic metal toxicity of having silver amalgams in your teeth. The holistic dentist I found at that time looked scary, but he did the job right. He removed those amalgams with a protective rubber cover, so I wouldn't swallow any of it during the procedure. My holistic doctor was taking care of me during that time and I was on a detox protocol to make the removal process as safe as possible. That protocol, which incorporated the doctor's recommendations and my own research, included vitamin C 3000mg daily, vitamin D 5,000IU daily, zeolite 3 dropperfuls daily, activated charcoal 2 capsules three times daily, bentonite magma 2 tablespoonful daily, liver support three times daily, and vitamin E 400IU once daily for 5 days. It was still not the smoothest process. There was fever, fatigue, joint pain, sensitivity to light, and other beautiful things associated with metal toxicity. But I was positive it would pass. I was patiently lying in bed for literally weeks afterwards. And it passed. I started feeling better and better every day. I believe this was a big step towards my healing, too.

As I was digging for more information, I realized what a toxic home we had. I tested the water and couldn't believe my eyes. The water filter came in the mail a few days later. I started reading every label on our beauty products and more than half ended up in the garbage, including baby shampoo. I replaced fluoride toothpaste with propolis toothpaste. The beautiful healing journey continued.

In my professional life, I was getting more and more shaky though. Here I was a graduate from a great school with a pharmacy degree, who's now shifting into natural medicine. Was it so weird? Now, I know it's not so unusual. My father had always pushed for natural methods, since I was a kid. I vividly remember him making a concoction of vitamin C and garlic when we were sick. My grandma had kombucha in her kitchen all the time, and she liked herbal teas for coughs. I fought these ideas during my first few years as a pharmacist. I would tell my family that we've advanced so much with medicine that there was no need for those silly natural and holistic methods. But then my illness turned me around. I am still the biggest believer in medicine, because for many health problems there's a strong need for it. But for chronic diseases that originate from poor dietary choices, toxicities, etc., there's a wonderful functional approach. For some that decide to take control, to get in the center of their healing, to get the self-management tools, there are beautiful complementary, functional, and integrative options that work.

So naturally the next step was to learn more about integrative healing options for myself. I have never stopped learning after becoming a pharmacist. I was taking courses for geriatric consultant certification and performing clinical consulting in the geriatric field, and training in something more holistic was the next step. When I read about functional medicine I almost jumped up with excitement. This was me! This was what I believed medicine should concentrate on! This became so much of an interest to me that I decided to get certified.

And that's when I found Dr. Kalish, his method and his clinical training. Later, I got certified as a functional medicine practitioner through his clinical training. I've seen many proactive clients in my practice that transformed completely.

I went on to graduate from a top school, the University of Florida, with a Doctor of Pharmacy degree. I always enjoyed being a pharmacist. I always felt bad for my very sick patients in the pharmacy who would come in over and over with a longer and longer list of medications. Being a chronic patient is not fun, and the fact that you picked up this book and are trying to change things for yourself is impressive and deserves respect. My best client is always a proactive client looking for self-management tools.

Unfortunately, not many websites were very informative when I was diagnosed. There were not many blogs, forums, or chats that had IBD communities. And forget about Facebook groups. They were nonexistent then. As much as I value the abundance of information out there, it also scares me. Just recently, on one Facebook group page I saw someone strongly recommending swallowing worms to get better. Would you try swallowing worms without medical supervision?

I've done so much research on IBD and I don't think I'll ever be done with it. I think this is the mission I'll carry on. I'd love to find ways to truly end IBDs and other digestive illness. I read medical literature and studies from the US and Europe on a regular basis. Functional medicine has more research to show now and there's so many options for Crohn's and colitis. The search for the root cause is very important when you are trying to figure out an individual chronic case, and now I apply all that knowledge in my client cases. Functional, complementary, and integrative methods don't just apply to Crohn's and colitis patients. The strategies are suitable for any immune system disorder like Celiac disease, ulcerative colitis, IBS, etc.

When I was experimenting with nutritional changes for a Crohn's disease diet, I had plenty of setbacks. Some of the food that you may think is the healthiest may cause inflammation and pain. For example, soy is still considered a "health food" but most IBD patients can't tolerate it. It's so important to know what foods cause your pain. It's important to keep a journal. I teach different ways to cool down inflammation with diet. Depending on each case, you may need to start with an elimination diet or go for a strict low-carb paleo or even a semi-vegetarian diet for a short period of time.

Many doctors won't agree with me here. Some gastroenterologists say that Crohn's patients can eat anything. I will give them a few more years to realize the importance of an anti-inflammatory diet. Anti-inflammatory diets, or healing diets, did work for me and my clients. I think it's important to find a doctor that you connect with. Be in the center of healing. Remember, you control your health. Draw up your healing vision board. Place yourself in the center point of the healing map and place all the practitioners around you—not you around them. It's your healing time. By drawing your healing gut map, choosing calm colors, placing positive images, and, most importantly, concentrating on the healing part instead of concentrating on the disease, you'll start to shift the energy toward healing.

My first clinical and practical steps of learning functional medicine included figuring out functional diagnostic tests. I was fascinated by how interesting it was to interpret them and after interpreting them, how much of a difference it made to fix those missing gaps for chronic patients. All functional medicine fixes can be complementary to traditional medicine; we can only make your condition better using an integrative approach. For example, you might be a patient on a medication that is working for your IBD. This medication has improved your condition, it has improved the inflammatory markers, and you are feeling better with fewer symptoms. Your therapy goal was achieved, but you started developing folic acid deficiency from methotrexate, B12 deficiency from PPIs like Prilosec or Prevacid, and felt exhausted. So often, supplementing will keep you in remission, yet *without* fatigue.

When I was doing my hormone testing and was still being mentored through clinical rounds, I felt like I wanted to write a love letter to my teacher. I didn't know that my period could be painless and not bothersome until I used functional medicine protocols. It was such an eye opener. I wanted to shout out loud, "Why won't other women use this too?" I was excited and feeling great. I want that for you. Feeling great can become your reality.

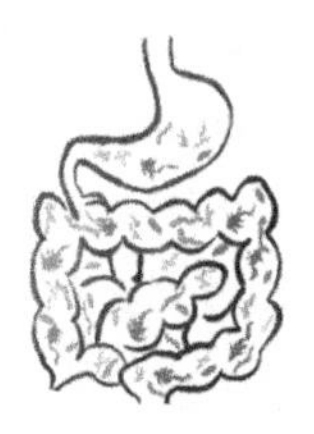

Chapter 2
TRIED EVERYTHING?

"Our bodies are our gardens,
to the which our wills are gardeners."
—William Shakespeare

By now you may feel like you've tried everything on earth to heal your IBD—or at least, many things. Traditional, alternative, complementary, scary ones, or maybe even some things I don't know about (which is unlikely, but not impossible). If you tried so many different things to improve, why haven't you healed yet? I ask my clients that question all the time. When I think about major obstacles for my clients and what prevents them from getting better, I find that dietary changes are one of their biggest problems. And I get that. If you've been eating the same way for thirty or forty years, it would be super hard to change. It seems like it's impossible to break those habits, but I know from my experience and from the experiences of my clients, that it is in fact doable, especially if you are feeling so sick that you can't think about anything else but being sick. That is the tipping point, the burning moment when you stop and understand that you are willing to do so much, to travel so far, to eat soil, to jump through any hoops, just to get relief. For those that have difficulties in breaking their habits, it really helps to use the mindfulness techniques I incorporate in my program.

Going on a gluten-free or dairy-free diet might sound challenging, but it can be done in baby steps, just like the hundreds of my clients that did it. Yes, many of them had a tough time in the beginning, but the moment they realized that they really could change their diet habits they suddenly felt their momentum of empowerment rising.

Maybe you are one of those people that have been there and done that with Crohn's/colitis and went through the doctor appointments, waited in line to see yet another specialist and listened to another opinion and thought that maybe, just maybe, this doctor will give you the answer you wanted to hear or maybe you could take a chance and travel to some amazing, famous clinic, and this time get a magic pill that's just for you and no one else. But, that doctor from that special clinic would probably still tell you the same diagnosis and give you the same treatment plan as the traditional doctors that you've seen before.

X-ray series, MRIs, colonoscopy preps, and other testing that requires you to go through very uncomfortable steps have most likely been part of your experience. Sometimes you can end up dehydrated, in more pain, but often hopeful, because if the test results find the cause of your problem, maybe the solution will be found as well.

You may have a story or two to share. One of my clients told me a story about how during her colonoscopy prep she had Jell-O the night before. She did the whole thing right. She only ate foods from her list and took the medication she was supposed to take, but she forgot about the "clear Jell-O only" rule for the colonoscopy, and had the red Jell-O instead. As you could imagine, the next thing you know the red Jell-O showed up on her colonoscopy looking like it was blood. And that's not a funny story at all, beside the fact that she needed to redo that colonoscopy. She was also scared for four weeks thinking she was bleeding heavily inside. Now it's possible to share these stories on Facebook, forums, and other social media, ask questions, and often get right answers.

What about your other searches for your possible root causes? If you've been dealing with Crohn's or colitis or any other digestive mess, I'm sure you've been doing some research about amalgams and mercury or other heavy metal poisoning that's associated with immune diseases like Crohn's or colitis.

Inflammatory bowel disease causes are unknown, and ever since I got into this topic years ago I've been constantly researching it. I even went for my doctorate in pharmacy to get better at reading clinical trials and researching papers and to be able to differentiate a quality study from a heavily sponsored one. I learned about clinical trials associated with Crohn's and colitis during the entire three years of school. Although there have been many advances with the class of drugs used for IBD (called biologicals), there aren't many new developments approved or new breakthrough drugs or traditional solutions for IBDs.

Since I love figuring things out, digging and researching, every client's case that came into my practice was very interesting work for me. It was like a great equation I just had to solve.

Some of the recent research associates the possible causes of Crohn's with microbiome changes (your gastrointestinal flora) and bacterial causes (like HPylori, etc.). The research is creating more space for additional studies dealing with antimicrobial use and some appropriate, quality probiotic use.

We don't know the clear-cut real causes for Crohn's or colitis, but many causes are being investigated and those include dietary habits, environmental influence, and stress hormones. The new testing technologies are now able to pick up on genetic variations that are associated with Crohn's and colitis and even traditional laboratories can test for them. Even if they found genetic variance associated with IBDs on the test, they still would not confirm that this was your root cause of Crohn's or colitis.

If you had someone with genetic markers for Crohn's/colitis and that person smoked for many years, lived in a polluted town, ate a Western diet and lived a stressful life compared to someone with the same Crohn's predisposition who ate well, included calming foods in their diet, lived in an environmentally clean town, exercised, didn't smoke, had a limited sugar intake and meditated daily, which one would have a faster trigger to get sick? It's possible that the one with the healthier life style would never ever know that they had a genetic predisposition to Crohn's or colitis, because no switch would ever turn on the disease.

Smoking was researched as a possible root cause by many studies.

You are probably aware that smoking is a major contributor to Crohn's. It's not considered the cause, but it is associated with severity of Crohn's and higher risk of having a Crohn's surgery. There are other risk factors, like ethnicity and age. The onset of the disease commonly starts in the thirties. I was also diagnosed in my thirties. Now I see young kids being diagnosed with it in their teens, and I so want this stopped so no kid has to suffer from the pain and embarrassment of this illness.

Although I understand how hard it is to quit smoking, I also know that it's worth living without symptoms. For ulcerative colitis, data doesn't find smoking to be a contributing risk factor, in fact its association with reduced exacerbations. But does that mean you need to go and start smoking? I've seen a client who did just that. He believed he had found a cure for his illness. Oh, the power of setting your mind to something.

The Role of Genetics in the Case of IBD

To this day, not all patients are getting genetic testing to confirm their predisposition for the disease. For example, the Prometheus IBD test is very accurate in telling Crohn's and colitis apart, as well as IBD vs. non-IBD conditions. Unfortunately, not many patients get genetic testing done to be more certain about the disease. And if you haven't yet done genetic markers testing, including testing inflammatory markers VEGF, ICAM, VCAM, CRP, SAA, as well as markers pANCA, anti-CBir1, anti-OMPC, DNAse sensitive pANCA and genetic (NOD2 variants SNPs 8, 12, 13), you may soon be able to get more information about your disease through those.

The advances in the field of genetics are amazing and I'm so proud to be a health care professional, but are people mentally ready to handle knowing all their genetic predispositions for all illnesses? There's

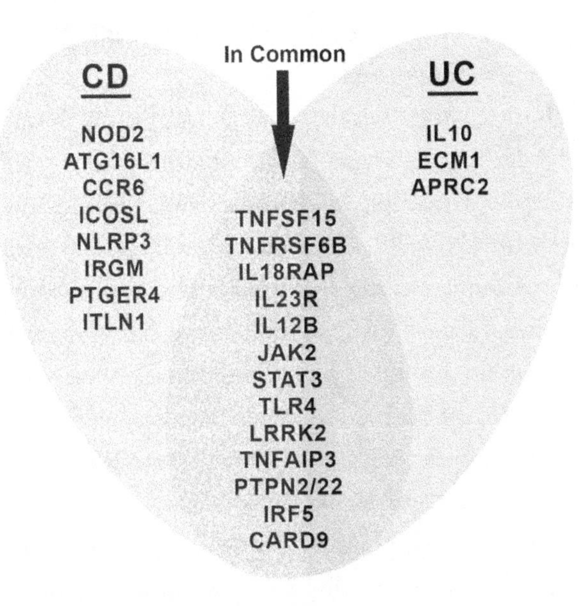

something about all genetic testing that I am concerned about. If in the future we will be able to test for all kind of genetic predispositions, how will people feel when they find out that they have a predisposition for a certain disease? It will definitely create concern and anxiety. It will make them worry to a point of physical ailment, hence a self-fulfilling prophecy. You may be curious why I am even bringing this up. There's a great point, I promise. If we understand that our emotional and mental health is directly related to our physical health on a deep level, we will also understand that healing a physical condition like Crohn's/colitis will need to involve emotional and mental health. The patient will respond to healing that much better, even with genetic issues.

Dietary Concerns as Possible Root Causes of Crohn's and Colitis

To this day it's not officially accepted that poor diet is the cause of Crohn's or colitis. Whether I am comfortable with that or not, we need to deal with reality. The reality is that many doctors are not trained to incorporate nutritional advice for IBDs, and that's where functional medicine becomes indispensable.

Although there are studies that associate Crohn's with certain dietary intake, it's harder for a study to be accepted on a large scale unless it's a real big study. For example, a retrospective Japanese study suggested that patients with Crohn's disease had higher intakes of sugar, fat, fish, and shellfish. A similar study from Israel also suggested a possibility of a dietary cause. Patients with Crohn's were eating more fatty foods, especially chemically modified fats and sugar. They also ate less fruits and had a lesser intake of fructose, potassium, magnesium, and vitamin C. Three large European studies suggested that, again, sugar was the problem. Sugar intake was significantly higher in Crohn's patients as compared to non-Crohn's groups. Can we safely say sugar intake could also be associated with Crohn's disease? Newer studies associated candida with Crohn's, which makes total sense to me. Years of inflammation from stress, causing leakiness of the gut, and eating too much sugar can lead to candida overgrowth with a possible result of an immune gut disease such as Crohn's or colitis.

If you tried different diets and had success for a short term and then didn't see results, it may not be because the diet didn't work. There could have been other factors that exacerbated the condition, like extra stress, hormone changes, medication switches, emotional triggers, and others. Don't give up when you are going for a true healing diet. With my clients, I try to give the basics of the diet in the beginning and continue with the nutritional changes slowly but surely. A recent study in the *Journal of Gastroenterology* from May 2015, confirms the suggestions that specific diets can be considered a cause and the treatment.

If you are a frequent visitor on IBD forums or blogs you may find quick fix few-week diets like gluten-free, dairy-free, soy-free, non-GMO, organic, no beer, no sugars, no spicy food, no nuts, no wine, no red meat, low residue, and others. All those may work, but it must be a systematic analysis-based approach. Just getting rid of the beer and continuing smoking and eating cheeseburgers every day may not necessarily work.

If you've been to more advanced blogs you may have seen diet options that were a bit more complicated and had more scientific research behind them, like specific carbohydrates diet, Low FODMAP diet, GAPS diet, and others. Those diets have worked for some of my clients, and they went into remission on those diets. Anti-inflammatory diets are not a one size fits all situation. If a diet trial didn't work, then the next step would be to move on to doing food allergy testing.

The Role of the Immune System in Cases of Crohn's Disease and Ulcerative Colitis

Although Crohn's and colitis are inflammatory bowel diseases associated with a malfunctioned immune system response, you would still want to know what gets triggered first. Triggers could be anything from good bugs overgrowing, pathogenic bacteria, inappropriate diet, an excess of sugar, chemicals, antibiotics, certain medications, stress, etc. Genetics also play a role here. There are certain genetic variances pertaining to Crohn's and certain ones that pertain to ulcerative colitis and there are those that pertain to both. Science is still undecided whether it's still just genetic related or genetic related that was triggered. The genetic markers that predispose the disease, causing the immune system to break down are influenced by unfavorable circumstances like the effect of environmental factors. Still, it's in our hands to improve some important factors like gut microbiome, clean diet, stress reduction, elimination of pathogens, and more, so the disease possibly never develops or goes into remission.

Environment and Pollution as Crohn's and Colitis Possible Root Causes

As mentioned previously, there are a few factors associated with these disorders: genetics, the immune system, and the environment. Antigens

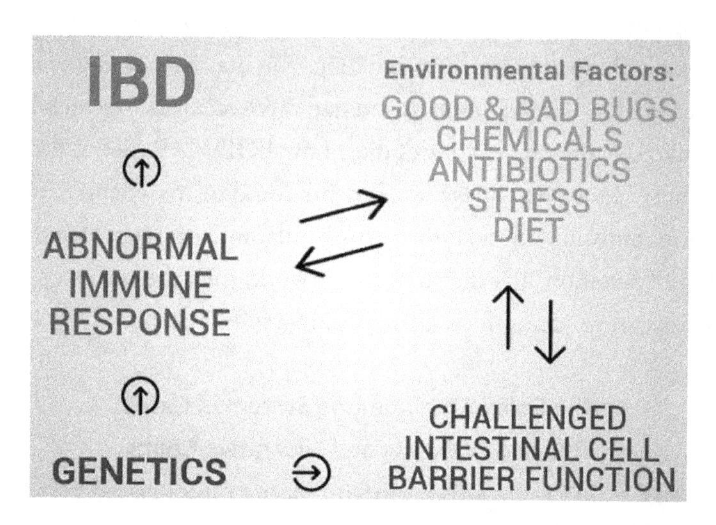

(foreign substances) are found in our environment. There is a possibility that our immune system overreacts to these foreign substances, causing inflammation.

Until very recently, European Jews and Caucasians made up most of the Crohn's cases in the US and in most industrialized countries. That's still true but changing. The European Commission observed that when the Asian population moved to urban-industrial societies of the West, their chances of getting Crohn's disease increased and were almost equal to the chances of people that already lived there. Now, we are getting more African-American IBD cases in North America and the United Kingdom.

Infections as Possible Root Causes of Crohn's and Colitis

When I was originally researching possible causes of Crohn's disease and read my first article about Mycobacteria, I got excited! Don't be surprised. I was happy because, if that was the true cause, it would be simple enough to eradicate Mycobacterium with a strong antimicrobial (antibiotic) and finally cure Crohn's disease. Mycobacterium avium subspecies paratuberculosis is a bacterium that's associated with tuberculosis and leprosy. It's also sometimes found in the gut flora of Crohn's patients, so naturally there have been more investigations on this topic. If you go to PubMed.com and search for this association, you can find numerous—but not very recent—studies and articles on it. Microbiome-associated research is certainly on the rise, and if this possible root cause is revisited and researched we may get more definitive answers. And I believe we are only at ground zero with gut microbiome research. We have yet to figure out what commensal bacteria species can be replaced for Crohn's/colitis patients in a way that they will survive the process and remain in the system. Oh, the wonders of modern medicine.

Birth Control as a Possible Association with Increased Risk of Developing Crohn's and Colitis

Since hormonal contraceptives were introduced to the market in the 1960s, the numbers of newly reported Crohn's patients have increased. A recent study published in 2017 in the *European Journal of Gastroenterology and Hepatology* confirms that the use of birth control or oral contraceptives is associated with higher risk for developing Crohn's and ulcerative colitis in a host that is originally genetically predisposed, meaning in a person that already had genetic markers for Crohn's and colitis. The use of birth control triggered the switch and caused the symptoms.

Association of Accutane with Crohn's and Colitis Cases

Some studies suggest that Accutane (generically called isotretinoin) can possibly cause IBDs, including Crohn's disease and ulcerative colitis. Now even a multi-million-dollar trial has ruled that Accutane is a probable cause. Thankfully, this cause is becoming obsolete, since the number of new Accutane prescriptions have decreased significantly.

Mercury and Other Heavy Metals as Possible Root Causes of IBDs

Documentations suggest that mercury fillings could poison the digestive system by slowly leaching out and accumulating in cells, tissues, joints, etc. Mercury is a heavy metal that can potentially become extremely toxic to our system. All this is not scientifically supported by medical studies. Nevertheless, I remove all of my mercury amalgams and did mercury detoxification with natural products.

Vitamin D Deficiency as a Possible Root Cause of IBDs

Having very low vitamin D levels is associated with many chronic conditions, including Crohn's disease. Vitamin D was shown to improve many chronic disease symptoms. Vitamin D has been researched and even scientifically proven to improve the symptoms of Crohn's disease. Functional medicine specialists, naturopathic doctors and holistic specialists started to raise awareness about symptoms of vitamin D deficiency and how important it was to have adequate vitamin D levels. It was about a decade after that when the traditional medicine community caught up with them in supporting those same studies. Well, better late than never! Research has shown that the bioactive form of vitamin D3 (1,25 dihydroxy vitamin D) can improve the symptoms of Crohn's disease. Now, it's common practice for doctors to write prescriptions for Vitamin D. Please, make sure it's vitamin D3 you are getting, not D2. Lots of research supports that vitamin D3 is at least twice as effective in raising vitamin D levels in the body, produces greater storage for vitamin D and converts to the active form faster. It is very important to test vitamin D levels periodically to stay in the optimum range between 50—80 ng/ml

Antibiotic Use and Overuse as a Possible Root Cause of IBDs

Another possible connection to Crohn's disease and colitis is over use of antibiotics. There is more research on the horizon for different methods on controlling Crohn's disease or colitis flare ups other than the use of antibiotics, but, in the meantime the treatment protocol suggests the use of antibiotics for flares because that's what seems to cool down those severe exacerbations. During or after antibiotic use, it's important to take probiotics in order to restore the normal gut flora that antibiotics have depleted.

Traditional Treatment Plans and Genotyping

Let's mention some traditional treatment options. I'm a pharmacist, after all! These include a few classes of drugs: anti-inflammatory agents, antibiotics, immunomodulators, anticholinergics for symptomatic relief of spasm pain, antidiarrheal and pain medications. Depending on where you are on the severity scale of the disease you may have already taken some of these medications like mesalamine, prednisone or biologicals. These come with a long list of serious side effects. The goal of traditional therapy is to put the patient into remission. But, how do you know if that patient will experience the side effects of that medicine or if that medicine is even appropriate for that patient to begin with? That is where genotyping comes into play. Genotyping is a method that can be used in assessing the risk or appropriateness of starting a medication regimen. For example, during a recent study using genotyping, researchers showed that you could prevent drug-related (in that case AZA azathioprine) pancreatitis in Crohn's patients that were carriers of the variant C allele gene. So, in the future, pharmacogenomics will become one of the most important factors in choosing one medication over another. Some doctors are already incorporating genotyping in their practice. Ask your doctor about genotyping and your pharmaceuticals.

Other Non-Conventional Treatment Options

There are also second-line medications like medical cannabis and LDN (low dose naltrexone). Some traditional doctors feel comfortable recommending these therapies. There's more large-scale research required to be able to assess the safety and efficacy of these treatments, but there are some positive studies for both. For example, there was a Norwegian study published in January of 2018 in the *Journal of Crohn's and Colitis* concluding that LDN initiation decreased the need for traditional medications.

If you are a Crohn's or colitis warrior who has been through surgeries like bowel resections, ileostomy, colectomy, and strictureplasty, you know how tough it is maintain a "normal" lifestyle, especially if you are left with a stoma. Looking at the bright side, the medicine and the surgeries are so advanced now that you can get back to "normal." And if you want to feel even better, there are more options for you.

Oral Health and IBDs

In functional medicine, gut health affects immune system health and that plays a role in many autoimmune diseases. We need to realize that digestion of food starts at the very top, in our mouth. Oral health is directly related to good gut health and having IBDs can directly affect oral health. Taking certain medications can cause dry mouth, acidic mouth, etc., creating room for unfavorable bacterial overgrowth. Simple solutions to keep your mouth healthy, besides proper tooth brushing, include flossing or water picking, eliminating processed sugars, using toothpaste without fluoride, gargling with water mixed with sea salt and even using probiotic toothpaste.

One cure fits all for IBDs?

I'm often asked what vitamins, minerals, or nutraceuticals work best for Crohn's/colitis. While that could be an entirely new book altogether, you need to realize that it's individually based. Ideally you want to work with a functional medicine specialist experienced with digestive illnesses to review your case for an individual recommendation. There are so many commonly used nutraceuticals in IBD that mostly address inflammation and immune system support. Probiotics have been used in Crohn's and colitis for decades with successful results. Patients with IBDs elect to try these natural medicines because of failed attempts with traditional methods. These agents are not just popular for Crohn's and colitis, but are also used for other conditions. Probiotics are living organisms of bacteria or yeast, and the most common ones include Saccharomyces boulardii, Lactobacillus, and Bifidobacteria. Probiotics are introduced as "friendly" recolonizing agents and often restore the flora for patients with IBDs. These would be the agents to use if a possible root cause of IBD is related to bacterial overgrowth in the gut. Most programs and natural therapies are never one size fits all. If you are looking to truly resolve each case, you should look into each case individually.

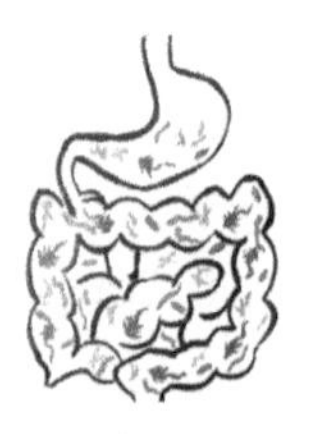

Chapter 3
FUNCTIONAL MEDICINE WORKS!

"There is more wisdom in your body than in your deepest philosophies."
– Friedrich Nietzsche

Other Options?

You know how important it is to find a healthcare specialist that has great communication with you. Even better is when your healthcare practitioner is familiar with complementary medicine and methods that work for your condition. Some functional medicine experts, like myself, emphasize the practice of creating a great therapeutic relationship with their clients in addition to researching the root cause of their illness, finding great integrative solutions and educating clients to be better at self-managing their health.

You will feel the connection with your specialist, and in many cases, it's an instant connection. You feel that instant shift of energy just by initiating and getting excited to start working with him or her. From my experience, it's very important to establish the trust, authority and that connection.

I love the phrase "functional medicine works," not only because I was able to heal completely using functional medicine, but also from my experience with my clients. "Functional medicine is the opposite of dysfunctional medicine," as one great functional medicine doctor says. Functional medicine treatments focus on the optimal functioning of the body and its organs, usually involving an integrative approach to health. There are great functional medicine diagnostics (saliva, dry urine, stool testing, and more) that will also uncover hidden root causes.

In functional medicine there's a great starting tool, the initial questionnaire. I take a full history as part of a root cause investigation for your wellness program. What does it mean to take a good first health history? That means that I ask you questions that maybe other health practitioners didn't have time for or were not trained to ask.

To functional medicine specialists, it's very important that I find out all the details of your emotional health, personality traits, your approach to stress, the way you react to things, and even how happy your childhood was.

Are you still carrying a lot of trauma? Were you exposed to chemicals when you were a child? All these questions are puzzle pieces for me, as a consultant, to put together.

For example, in my case, in 1986 there was a catastrophic nuclear explosion at an atomic station in Chernobyl. I lived in a town that was close enough for that radiation to affect me. At that time, I was only 12 years old and being that young it had an even greater impact on my health. At that age the hormones are changing, the detoxification system is affected, and the thyroid needs lots of support. My health was affected.

Giving this type of information on my initial questionnaire would give a great clue to a functional medicine specialist.

For others, it could be variations of different toxicities. It could be a chronic exposure to mold, or exposure to paint or other chemicals that are related to acetone. The key here is to be very thorough.

It's important to get an overall health picture. It's even important to include where you were physically born and raised for the purposes of nutritional recommendations.

Ideally, you want to list all the supplements you're taking during your initial consult. To me, as a pharmacist, that becomes of great importance. There are many drug—herb interactions, which can go unnoticed because supplements are still not a part of the medication profile in many clinics and many pharmacies. That's where the interaction can get overlooked.

We also need to know your food allergies and food sensitivities. Even if you are just a little uncomfortable after eating bread or get a rash or have diarrhea after eating pizza, definitely report it. Some patients don't pay attention to any reactions because they do not know there could be an association between food and illness.

Keeping a journal is a great tool to figure out reactions and excessive bowel movement after certain foods. Also, discuss your food cravings with your specialist. That information really matters. If you tend to crave sweets, this sometimes indicates a possibility of having candida overgrowth, blood sugar instability or adrenal or hormone problems.

As our lengthy interview gets us closer to finding your root cause, it is possible for both the practitioner and the patient to have an "A-ha" moment where it becomes clear what your original root cause was.

Quite often in functional medicine, liver support is initially recommended for a better liver phase 1 and phase 2 support. Liver support is a gentle way of helping this large detoxification organ move out toxins more efficiently. In that case the protocol often includes milk thistle, glutathione, methylated folate, glycine, and others. The reason behind starting liver support is that many chronic digestive disease patients have a problem with detoxification.

Liver support can also be addressed with a certain healing diet which includes lots of artichokes, blueberries, raspberries, avocado, cruciferous vegetables, fatty, wild, omega fish, and liver-supporting teas like roasted dandelion or milk thistle. Ideally, you want to first choose foods that promote liver support. During your time of liver support supplementation, you also want to be careful with foods that are toxic, such as processed sugars, processed oils, fried foods, artificial additives, preservatives, and soda. Avoiding them is extremely important because you don't want to be adding chemicals at the same time that you are removing them. You also want to avoid foods that are genetically modified because in some complicated cases they can trigger an immune reaction and Crohn's/ colitis patients have a problem with their immune system to begin with.

It's no surprise that many Crohn's/ colitis patients have trouble digesting food proteins. Avoiding gluten, dairy, and soy proteins can have that wonderful effect of cooling down inflammation. If you are up for a challenge you can even start an elimination diet which often saves you money on food allergy testing. With the kick-start of liver support and an elimination diet we get an additional effect of decreasing that inflammation.

At some point in our long interview or initial consultation we could also figure out your genetic predisposition for diseases. But our job isn't to dwell on your genetic predisposition, since we can't do much about it; our job is to make sure the trigger isn't there to inflame it. If a patient is living a stress-free life, eating a healing diet or eating generally well, and living in an environment that's not toxic, they may never know that they are genetically predisposed to a certain illness, because the trigger was never fired.

Testing for genetic predispositions is also a catch twenty-two. It's great to find out certain details from the test when you have something to fix the problem with, but, if you just find a problem without any solution for it, then it can get more stressful.

Lifestyle interventions are very important for healing and a great wellness plan incorporates nutraceuticals, lifestyle modifications, meditation, dietary changes, and other aspects into your life. If underlying stress isn't addressed, it may take much longer to heal. Basic tools of displacing stress perception, as well as decreasing emotional reactions to stress, are very useful at this part of the program. These include EFTs, meditations, breathing techniques, NLP, and more.

In functional medicine we customize the program for every individual case so it's best to work with a professional guide. Crohn's and colitis patients are perfect for this type of healing modality because they often have uncovered root causes that need to be addressed. For my chronic digestive clients, I used a functional medicine program mostly adopted from great professionals in the field of functional medicine and science-based protocols. I also incorporate a few herbal antimicrobial protocols from science-based research. The program is also modified with my pharmacy-based knowledge and experience as a Crohn's patient to solve most cases of digestive problems.

As you start having fun with a healing diet, we start to work with functional diagnostics. There are many lab companies out there now and many of them are very credible. You can even order some lab tests on your own, bypassing the specialist, but you'll soon realize you can't get around needing help from someone to translate the results for you.

For example, in my program I like to use Bio health or DUTCH for adrenal/hormonal/neuroendocrine systems, and I like to use Diagnostic Solutions for stool testing, since they have PCR technology. DUTCH testing is adding other elements now, like neurotransmitters and organic acid testing, which makes it a very comprehensive functional diagnostic.

When testing your stool sample, we are not just looking for parasitic pathogens, bacterial pathogens, viral pathogens, H Pylori, normal flora, phyla microbiota, overgrowth bacteria, potential immune triggers, fungi, yeast, and parasites. We are also looking into digestion markers, inflammation markers, leaky gut markers, and even antibiotic resistance genes/phenotypes. All these markers are important when we are planning our recommendations for healing your intestines by decreasing inflammation, removing pathogens, adding healing programs, and recolonizing with probiotics. And the healing process continues.

When you address inflammation, you can't really bypass adrenal system support since balancing adrenals helps cool down the inflammation as an initial basic step. With Crohn's and colitis there's a lot of inflammation to be addressed! We do that often with herbal supplements. Adrenal support wellness plans often include adaptogen herbs, DHEA, pregnenolone, licorice root, or others.

Understand, while nutraceuticals are not pharmaceutical drugs, they still need to be monitored by a health care practitioner. For example, taking licorice root and having high blood pressure is not a good mix. This type of supplement interaction with a disease state needs to be recognized and addressed properly.

Once adrenal function is improved, gut pathogens are eliminated, and flora is reseeded with good bacteria using appropriate probiotics, it's time to investigate more. And investigating more is also individual. In some cases, the improvement from adrenal/hormonal balance and GI healing is so profound that there's no need to continue digging for more. In cases where symptomatic improvement is still very necessary, more digging is required. There are options with neurotransmitter testing, organic acid testing, and, depending on each case, even micronutrient testing. Sometimes diarrhea can be addressed with a neurotransmitter balance of dopamine, serotonin, tyrosine or others. There are documented Crohn's case studies by Dr. Hinz from NeuroResearch and studies researching how to fix gut bacteria that produce neurotransmitters and command neuroactivity.

Looking into OAT (organic acid testing) can be the next step in digging for a possible root cause. OAT functional testing is like a toxicity map. Looking into OAT results we can see what markers are associated with the possibility of candida overgrowth or issues with your mitochondria, which is huge and very important for healing. Without mitochondria properly functioning you cannot expect energy, and you will age prematurely. Without feeding the mitochondria the right nutrients, you can't expect the mitochondria to work for you.

If there's still a need for more testing—if, for example, the symptoms have improved but you are not yet fully at your goal—you can go with micronutrient testing. I find this test to be important. Not too many of my clients go through this test because by this point they feel so much better and they feel that there is no need for it. Nevertheless, replenishing missing nutrients can be the final key to energy and vitality. It's no surprise to find depletions in Crohn's/colitis patients because of chronic inflammation and absorption problems.

Restoring micronutrients can become essential for healing. For example, if you replenish B-vitamins, (and I mostly recommend active B-complex, just in case you are a poor metabolizer) for those who are completely depleted it would make a world of a difference for their sleep, energy, and even mood.

If you have sensitivities, respiratory problems, rashes, mood disorders, severe brain fog or others, then you may want to consider metal toxicity testing. These symptoms and others can be associated with having heavy metal toxicity in your system. Personally, I got rid of all of my mercury amalgams (silver fillings) because I read plenty of studies that associated having mercury with having Crohn's disease or IBDs—although, I'm not citing one particular study here or recommending you doing what I did. All I'm trying to do is to educate you and empower you to make your best health related decisions for yourself. I took out my amalgams because I just wanted to do everything

I had to do to heal, and not to ever say I didn't try something until I went into full remission. Whatever I had to do and try, I went for it. The process of taking out mercury amalgams wasn't easy. If you choose to remove silver fillings, consider going to an experienced biological dentist like a holistic dentist who has specialized tools in the mercury removal protocol. It's possible to feel sick afterwards, because when you go through metal detoxification, you can feel feverish, nauseous, shaky, and very uncomfortable. That happens because a heavier flood of mercury is now being pulled through your system and needs to be removed with the help of the liver, our major filter organ. It's important to drink a lot of water and fluids during this process and make sure that your elimination goes well. Sometimes that means taking a magnesium supplement or even stool softener. At this time, it's wise to do a support protocol because your immune system, your liver and your lymphatic system need extra care. That includes vitamin E, alpha lipoic acid, zeolite, activated charcoal, bentonite magma, liver support, high doses of liposomal or bioflavonoid vitamin C, vitamin E, vitamin D, and colostrum.

If the liver is not doing a great job at clearing toxins, then it will not help with the metal detox. You won't be able to clear the metals. If you're not going to the bathroom at least once or twice daily, you might reconsider doing metal removal because, if you do, you will pull metals from the system, but your body wouldn't be able to get rid of them, so you would reabsorb them and dump them back into your bloodstream, making you feel even sicker. Working with a professional expert that understands many aspects of detoxification is advisable.

When we heal digestive diseases in functional medicine we also want to look into thyroid health to rule out under active thyroid or other issues. Having a healthy thyroid relates to healthy adrenals and often means not much inflammation. Also, the opposite is true. If your thyroid is not performing well that means something could be going on with your hormones where adrenals are involved and inflammation becomes inevitable.

For those clients who like to figure out their food allergies or intolerances there are many labs available like ALCAT and MRT. These are pricey labs, so I always recommend going with an elimination diet first. Sometimes the results of food allergy testing may be very dietary restrictive, and the recommendations aren't always easy to follow. I've seen plenty of struggles, but it's not impossible. Sometimes finding out a food allergen can be a blessing. It can be that simple. One food that you removed from your diet, which you never expected to be a severe allergen, will now get you de-flamed.

After all this work with your functional medicine practitioner mentioned so far, your regular doctor may get pleasantly surprised with your diagnostics like inflammatory marker reduction, your iron level restoration, and the fact that your overall health picture is looking so much better. There's a chance some doctors may consider a reduction of drug therapy and even discontinuation of certain medications.

Functional medicine programs require a lot of patience, good intentions, and a lot of positive thoughts. They require your participation with full determination and excitement because that state of belief will carry you through those challenging days.

When you are in a program, working with me or another expert, every step of the way, you feel the guidance you need. You don't feel left alone at any point. You're given recommendations and support. The key is to empower yourself with recipes, tools for a positive state of mind and the step-by-step process to heal that I am sharing. And yes, functional medicine works.

I want to reflect on the quote by Friedrich Nietzsche in the beginning of this chapter: "There is more wisdom in your body than in your deepest philosophies." And I would like to ask you to give your body the chance to use its wisdom.

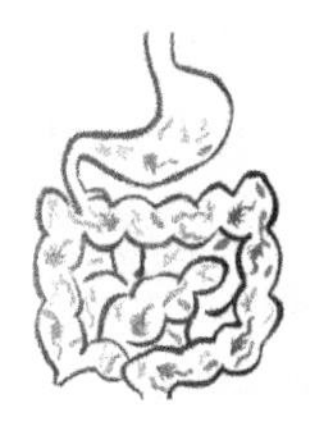

Chapter 4

FUNCTIONAL SOLUTIONS: FUNCTIONAL DIAGNOSTICS, TESTING FIRST?

"Health is not simply the absence of sickness."

– Hannah Green

Have you tried that?

Functional medicine testing options are now growing. More and more labs are offering saliva, stool, urine, blood, dry urine, hair and other testing. The reason you want to invest in functional diagnostics is because it will give you more opportunity to see what else could possibly be wrong. You will see and take advantage of the opportunity to find the root cause of a problem. Functional diagnostic testing can give you more options to figure things out.

Neuroendocrine/Adrenal/Hormonal Functional Testing

- What the test does: This type of test helps your functional medicine expert figure out what adrenal support is best in your case in order to address your inflammation.
- Who should get it: Any Crohn's and colitis patient with inflammation and fatigue.
- Tips on getting the testing: Some quality functional diagnostic labs are mentioned in this book in the resource chapter.

The first test you usually want to consider is the neuroendocrine test, or, as we call it, adrenal testing. Thankfully there are different ways to test adrenals. There is saliva testing and now a newer option using dried urine.

Adrenal hormones are sometimes referred to as stress hormones. When you have stress for too long, hormones are eventually affected. Our stress response can eventually break down or get impaired and trigger female sex hormone imbalance and gut imbalance with all its digestive symptoms.

Cortisol is one of the major stress hormones produced by the adrenal glands. The adrenal glands play a very important role in the inflammatory process. Cortisol also regulates blood pressure and controls blood sugar. It is very important in the metabolism of carbohydrates, fats, and proteins. Cortisol is normally secreted as a response to stress in the body, whether the stress is physical, dietary, emotional, chemical, or psychological. Because of the cortisol being secreted in response to the stress, it can lead to breakdown of muscle protein. In the liver, it can also convert amino acids into energy.

Cortisol is responsible for making energy from the glycogen that's normally stored as glucose or sugar in the liver. When there's chronic stress, the body continually produces cortisol. At some point the adrenals will have a difficult time producing cortisol because they will eventually be weakened and exhausted. This is sometimes referred to as adrenal burnout. This can cause the body to store more fat and experience more fatigue and more depression, as well as other symptoms of chronic digestive problems.

DHEA is another hormone produced by the adrenal glands that is responsible for many important functions of the body. When we're not stressed, cortisol and DHEA remain stable and balanced. When we're chronically stressed, DHEA is disturbed and it cannot be converted properly. Often DHEA has a broken conversion to estrogen because of chronic stress.

At the same time, if the body is under stress, pregnenolone hormone (which is synthesized in the adrenal glands) will re-route and divert to produce cortisol, which lowers progesterone. Low levels of progesterone make a very messed up case of hormone imbalance! I speak from experience.

When the entire hormone balance system is out of whack it sometimes becomes beneficial to use DHEA and pregnenolone as supplementation. It's extremely important to take DHEA and pregnenolone properly because in unregulated amounts they can cause side effects. Looking at the lab results of the adrenal testing such as saliva or dry urine would be the way to go first before using these potent supplements.

Now it's becoming popular to use cortisol-boosting supplements or adrenal supplements, and there's a lot of them on the market. Some people are trying out adrenal supplements without success, which isn't surprising because they don't know what their dose should be.

Many are asking what Cortisol Awakening Response (CAR) is and why it's important in the testing of adrenals. CAR is a predictable rise and fall of cortisol within the first hour of awakening. The result of the CAR can also help you interpret how the value relates to how you are feeling.

This data gives you a much better picture of what's happening in the entire adrenal system, and, more specifically, it gives you a picture of how stress in that person is contributing to poor health in general and poor digestive health particularly.

Who should do an adrenal test? Anyone with chronic stress. Maybe the better question is who should not be doing the test?

Elevated cortisol values after adrenal testing could mean that a patient is in an acute state of stress. Having a flare of Crohn's/colitis could put you in an acute state of stress which will make your cortisol levels rise. Acute stress lasts a short time and even a flare can be considered chronic stress since the stress on the body never stopped. This concept can be tricky. We must understand and look at other symptoms in a patient's history to see the causes of inflammation in the case of IBD. There could be other issues affecting the patient: emotional issues, glycemic control, unstable blood sugar. Over-exercise sometimes is a problem. Situations like these can explain higher levels of cortisol.

If the levels of cortisol on the HPA stress profile are all low, that is often the case in chronic stress caused on the HPA Axis to down-regulate and decrease the effect of too much cortisol. So, this is a post-effect, many IBD patients would show low values of cortisol on their adrenal testing.

With the low values of cortisol, we also need to rule out co-infections or gut infections in any chronic patient since they also promote further inflammation. Cortisol is a powerful anti-inflammatory steroid, and inflammation in the case of a patient with Crohn's/colitis could be triggering the HPA Axis to increase cortisol to decrease inflammation. After a while that becomes something that the HPA Axis cannot fulfill, and the levels of cortisol are now reduced.

The key here is to remove the sources of chronic inflammation and investigate possible gut infections and other triggers that might be causing this response. The second thing, ideally, is to give good nutrient support because you often find a Crohn's/colitis patient with a deficiency of vitamins, micronutrients, and antioxidants or maybe even omega-3 fats. Replenishing the nutritional deficiencies will help decrease the inflammation. Dietary anti-inflammatory improvements can also help with weight regulation and improve blood sugar regulation.

Some herbs that are used in the kitchen can decrease inflammation. These include cinnamon, turmeric, cloves, ginger, and rosemary. That could become an inexpensive anti-inflammatory help.

There is also a way of testing adrenal hormones through dry urine testing. The advantage of this testing is that with dry urine you are able to see the metabolites that are often the key to figuring out estrogen, progesterone, DHEA and cortisone values.

Correcting hormone imbalances according to the result of saliva testing or dry urine testing can decrease inflammation, balance sex hormones, and reduce the symptoms associated with inflammation, like pain, weight gain or weight loss. It can also help with female menopausal symptoms or PMS symptoms. The ovaries secrete estrogen, which is also produced by the adrenal glands and fat tissues, and that's why menopausal women really do benefit from this balance.

When there is chronic stress, in cases like Crohn's/ colitis or other digestive diseases, there is more demand for cortisol and DHEA. That comes at the expense of producing progesterone. That effect is heightened by an initial increase of cortisol and this normally drops the estrogen of mid-life menopausal women.

Stool Testing

- What the test does: This test uncovers possible bacterial pathogens, parasites, etc. with a goal to eliminate bad bacteria and replace good bacteria.
- Who should get it: Most people with gastrointestinal issues, especially Crohn's and colitis patients.
- Tips on getting the testing: See the resource chapter.

Testing stool with a good PCR technology testing company can uncover hidden root causes.

The newer testing technology will investigate many aspects of gut infections such as bacterial infection, parasitic infection, and others. They will investigate bacteria and viruses, such as E. Campylobacter, salmonella, Yersinia enterococlitica or others. There are also parasitic pathogens that you'd want to test for. Examples of those would be Giardia, Entamoeba histolytica, and Cryptosporidium. You want to make sure that the opportunistic bacteria are not overgrowing (the ones that are normally present in your gut). You want to make sure that those bacteria are not present in high or large amounts, because if you have an overgrowth, you may have the symptoms of dysbiosis. You don't want to have parasites because they can create an inflammatory atmosphere. Some people can be symptomatic while others do not present with symptoms and can act as a source for hidden inflammation.

A good PCR stool test will also test for inflammatory markers, gliadin markers, enzymatic production markers, immune system markers, and more. They will test for leaky gut markers like zonulin, fecal occult blood, and more. Interpreting a lab called GI map, for example, is really like looking into a map of your gut.

Organic Acid Test

OAT and micronutrient testing are very important in functional diagnostic testing for any chronic condition.

- What the test does: OAT and micronutrient testing can help figure out the missing nutrients that can improve detoxification, metabolism, immune system health, and more.
- Who should get it: Anyone who is exposed to toxins and/or has a chronic condition.
- Tips on getting the testing: See resources chapter.

Organic acids are metabolic intermediates produced in pathways of central energy production, detoxification, and testing on microbial activity, or neurotransmitter breakdown.

Accumulation of organic acids can be detected in urine and sometimes it signals metabolic inhibition or blocking. That metabolic blocking could be due nutrient deficiency, toxin build-ups, drug effects, or genetic enzyme deficit.

Organic acid testing is a nutritional test that can provide information from a single urine sample, and we can observe the following indicators:

1. Markers being high for bacteria or yeast overgrowth.
2. Methylation, sufficiency or insufficiency.
3. Neurotransmitter metabolites out of range indicating gut problems.
4. Phase one and phase two detoxification markers out of range.
5. Functional vitamin and mineral status that requires attention.
6. Functional B complex need.
7. Mitochondria production, a big problem with patients that have chronic digestive stress.
8. Other markers out of balance.

Correcting those can also help with energy problems in chronic disease patients. Nutritional deficiencies commonly found in patients with IBD are:

- Folic Acid
- Magnesium
- Vitamin B12
- Calcium
- Niacin
- Vitamin D

- Thiamine
- Zinc
- Vitamin K

Neurotransmitter Testing (NT)

- What the test does: This test can help figure out how to balance neurotransmitters better which will result in improvements of chronic conditions, mood, diarrhea, etc.
- Who should get it: People with chronic conditions, especially IBD patients where you can address specific symptoms with a general NT balance.
- Tips on getting the testing: See resources chapter.

The next testing is a neurotransmitter one, since patients with Crohn's and colitis often have mood disorders as a result of gut inflammation. This may also be from the pain, stress, malabsorption of nutrients, or other root causes.

Neurotransmitters are brain chemicals and they make sure that there's a good transmission of signals coming from one neuron to the next across synapses. Neurotransmitters work with certain receptors in the brain to affect and regulate a variety of processes like mental performance, pain response, energy, and emotions.

Functioning mostly in the central nervous system, neurotransmitters are chemical messengers of the brain. They communicate in the body's glands, organs, and muscles. Studies have shown that insufficient number of neurotransmitters can influence overall health and mood.

Certain neurotransmitters are associated with major conditions like adrenal dysfunction, hormonal imbalances, mood disorders, loss of mental focus, cognitive fog, loss of appetite, insulin resistance, addiction, and dependency.

So, looking at the symptoms of, for example, Crohn's patients, we realize that since there have been all kinds of digestive nutrient absorption problems, it's very possible to also have a neurotransmitter imbalance. Looking at neurotransmitters for a chronic digestive patient can help determine another root cause and correcting the neurotransmitter imbalance can improve symptoms of depression, as well as symptoms of loss of appetite, cognitive fog, and other related ones. Fixing neurotransmitter imbalance can also help with fatigue.

Balancing neurotransmitters can improve insomnia, energy, sexual dysfunction, and depressed mood.

The next test that would be great to look into would be…

Micronutrient Testing

It wouldn't be a big surprise to see deficiency of micronutrients in patients with digestive problems because there is an absorption issue in gut inflamed patients.

- What the test does: This is a blood test, which can figure out what micronutrients are missing.
- Who should get it: Patients with chronic conditions, fatigue, who are on medications that deplete micronutrients, etc.
- Tips on getting the testing: See resources chapter.

Having low amounts of certain nutrients can cause a chain reaction and micronutrient testing would include testing for vitamins like A's and B's, vitamins C, D, and K. It would include minerals like calcium, magnesium, manganese, zinc, and copper, and amino acids like glutamine, cyanine, fatty acids, antioxidants, CoQ10, vitamin E, and selenium, etc. It would also test for carbohydrate metabolism, for chromium, fructose sensitivity, glucose insulin sensitivity, and metabolites like choline and carnitine. Learning this information that pertains to insulin sensitivity, choline and correcting the problem can also be useful for women who have PCOS symptoms.

Being proactive and testing for micronutrient deficiencies can drastically change the way a patient feels if you replenish something that's been missing. Looking into micronutrient testing is something very useful in cases of so called sub-optimal vitamin D. As mentioned earlier, vitamin D deficiency is associated with chronic conditions, including IBDs.

Having a sub-optimal vitamin level doesn't automatically scream, "replenish" the vitamin or mineral. But if it's done, it often makes a very big difference in the way the patient feels, especially for inflammation.

Testing for Metals, Molds or Environmental Testing

This is another way to check out the possible root causes.

- What the test does: This is another way to check out possible root causes. These hair, urine or blood tests can show if there are dangerous metal levels in your system.
- Who should get it: Patients with chemical sensitivities, rashes, chronic conditions, severe fatigue, etc.
- Tips on getting the testing: See resources chapter.

Toxic body burden can be an accumulation of chemicals through our food, our environment, and the air we breathe. This accumulation, for some patients, can become a major problem, a major health-related issue, and it could trigger an autoimmune or neural degenerative disease, diabetes, or cancer. It's associated with constant exposure to environmental toxins. Some research suggests that if the exposure has been in the very early part of life, it could become worse for the patient.

It's known that newborn babies, unfortunately, are born with toxins and chemicals already in their system, because a lot of them come through the placenta in vitro. Environmental working group (EWG) works with numerous toxic compounds and found that over 200 of those toxic compounds were found in the cord blood of newborns. So, we must learn this information, evaluate it, and analyze it while making up a good functional medicine wellness program for you.

There are ways to test for toxins and metals, including hair tests, urine tests, blood tests, and more. Heavy metals are very difficult to address with treatments, but they should still be tested for because knowing the actual root cause could clear up the health picture.

Food Sensitivity Testing

- What the test does: This test measures the changes in certain cells to see allergic reaction to food.
- Who should get it: Anyone suspecting a strong food allergy or trying to figure out every possible root cause.
- Tips on getting the testing: See resources chapter.

There are a lot of immunological problems associated with food sensitivities. Food sensitivities are directly associated with inflammatory reactions in the system since it involves the cytokines and the white blood cells. If there's an infection or an injury, more cytokines are released. The more cytokines are released, the more inflammation. Food sensitivities are not yet completely understood, but they are not like food allergies. With food sensitivities we often have an IgG mediated immune response while a food allergy is often an immediate IgE mediated immune reaction and could possibly be life-threatening. While food sensitivity isn't life threatening, having low-grade inflammation from the chronic attack of the offensive food particles could become very damaging over time.

Looking into a food sensitivity test can be an "A-Ha" moment in functional diagnostic analysis. First it lets you know which foods you cannot tolerate. Secondly, if that food intolerance list is very long it may mean you have a problem with leaky gut.

The mediator release, which is like a reaction from the food that you're not tolerating, is the key event that leads to reaction. There are a few different food allergy/sensitivity testing technologies used to measure the changes in lymphocytes, monocytes, neutrophils, and eosinophils. The changes after food or a food chemical challenge are measured and reported as "reacted," "mildly reacted," or "none reacted." This list of foods can be used to put together a suitable diet and is a great strategy for creating a rotation diet..

I have some concerns about food intolerance testing, especially the IgG based testing. It's almost like opening a can of worms—patients avoid lots of foods because of the test and see no results. The problem is avoiding many foods which results in decrease of food diversity in the diet. This can have devastating effects on the gut microbiome due to depletion of numerous unique nutrients.

IgG informs you that your system is familiar with a certain food and if you tolerate it or not. The elimination diet may be a much cheaper (free) option to test for food intolerance accurately. Some testing companies use fresh cells instead of IgG which enables them to measure the total amount of inflammation in whole blood for the food in question. IgG antibody testing measures antibodies, not inflammation.

Putting It All Together

Analyzing every test is one extremely important step in the process. Your qualified functional medicine specialist can work out a proper testing sequence for you. It's very important to do the right kind of sequence. You don't want to start, for example, with organic acid testing if a patient is not even absorbing amino acids to be able to test them. You don't want to possibly do a heavy metal test in the beginning, either because the patient needs a lot of inflammatory support or adrenal support, or both.

So, having the right guidance here will be very important. But all these tests can become very valuable in addressing root causes of a chronic digestive condition.

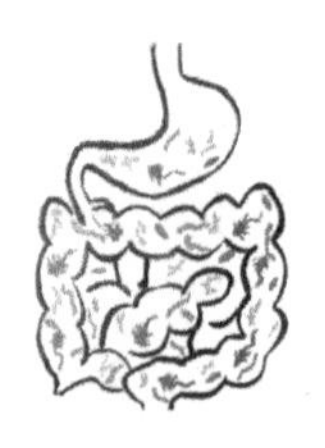

Chapter 5

FUNCTIONAL SOLUTIONS: ADRENALS, HORMONES AND GUT CONNECTION

"The secret of health for both mind and body are not to mourn for the past, not to worry about the future… but to live the present moment wisely and earnestly."
– **Siddhartha Gautama Buddha**

What Is the Relationship between Adrenals and Chronic GI Problems?

Adrenal glands are found atop the kidneys and are responsible for many functions. Adrenal health has started getting attention lately for a good reason. The adrenal glands are very important for our stress response, sex hormones, blood pressure regulation, cardiovascular health, and the metabolism of carbohydrates, fats and proteins. Adrenal dysregulation can be caused by different types of stressors, like dietary stress, work-related stress, environmental, chemical stress, gastrointestinal stress, emotional stress, lack of sleep, physical stress, and more. Chronic, unaddressed stress puts the body into constant burnout, causing dysregulation of the adrenal hormones, including cortisol.

Cortisol is that "feel good" hormone which you need for all basic bodily functions. Cortisol or glucocortisol receptors are found in almost every cell of the body.

If you find yourself relying on coffee, sugar, or other stimulants to get through the day, then balancing your adrenals may be very beneficial for you. The initial step to balancing them is to start a well-balanced diet that's low in sugar, containing quality protein, quality fat, and lots of vegetables. Adrenal testing would be the next step in taking care of those glands so that inflammation can be addressed as well.

Why is the HPA Axis so important for adrenal/gut health?

It is a set of direct influencers and reactions between three major components. One is the hypothalamus. The second one is the pituitary gland. And the third one is the adrenal gland. The HPA Axis is the important connection between the central nervous system and endocrine system. And of course, it involves the adrenal glands.

What kind of relationship is there between stress hormones and the gut?

First, recent studies indicate that the gut microbiome, or gut flora, can affect the development and regulation of HPA Axis. Some of you know that our gut is our second brain—or our brain is our second gut. The gut and the brain are connected through the original development of the embryo cells. The brain and the gut send signals to control metabolism, immune system, and permeability. The brain depends on the normal floral or gut microbiota's functionality to make certain neurotransmitters. Although this connection between the gut and the brain is still being studied extensively, we now realize that mood can very much be dependent on what we are eating, how we are digesting, and how much we are assimilating nutrients.

We also know that chronic stress will result in intestinal permeability, which we call leaky gut syndrome. It is associated with low-grade inflammation, and now we are linking that to psychiatric disorders like depression. Having depression associated with Crohn's or colitis, having pain and diarrhea and other symptoms, can all be related to the imbalance of neurotransmitters, the same ones that affect the brain, as mentioned previously. And now we are also connecting to the neurotransmitters and the gut with a brain axis and chronic stress.

Normally produced lactobacillus and bifidobacteria in the gut produce GABA, which is a gama-aminobutyric acid. This is an important neurotransmitter in the brain. So, if something is going on in the gut that's making an overgrowth of normally present lactobacillus or bifidobacterium, the result may be low levels of certain neurotransmitters, and therefore brain related symptoms.

Gut microbiota interacts with the brain through different mechanisms, and as a result brain synapses can also alter microbiota of the gut. Both systems affect each other as a result.

We don't usually think that digestive and hormonal systems are connected, but any type of inflammation in the digestive system can initially cause increased production of cortisol, which is an anti-inflammatory hormone. The result would be damage in the intestinal lining, impairing the absorption of micronutrients that are extremely important. So, a direct result of digestive chronic inflammation can be the cause for hormone imbalance, and vice versa.

There are many patients who have digestive problems who also have hormone problems as a result, and we also have patients that have their hormones affecting their gut. People are often not familiar with what constant stress can do to their hormones, so addressing stress would be crucial. Stress can be physical, psychological, chemical, environmental, etc.

Gluten sensitivity sometimes causes inflammation—we call it silent inflammation. It can damage the tissues in the digestive tract, and it could also become a low-grade infection as a result of the initial chronic inflammation. It can also cause bloating, constipation, diarrhea, and, over the years, if there is moderate gluten intolerance, it can cause severe fatigue, weight gain, or depression. These symptoms can be uncomfortable for some, but some don't connect it to having gluten intolerance. The most well-known connecting hormone between the gut and the brain is called serotonin. It's used in anti-depressant medications.

The majority of serotonin is made in the gut, while only five percent of serotonin is produced in the brain. So, having damage in the gut from stress, gluten intolerance, chemicals, or gut infections can cause serotonin levels to be super low and therefore result in depression or mood changes.

Adrenal Hormones and Chronic Stress.

We all have stress in our lives and some of it we can't do anything about. If we are physically and emotionally exhausted and it's not being addressed with stress-reducing techniques, we end up getting sick. Stressors such poor diet, lack of sleep, chemical toxicity, co-infections, anxiety, and fears all cause chronic conditions, and we could say that many chronic conditions are caused by one or a combination of these stressors. Some people naturally perceive and handle stress well. Others don't have the techniques, the tools, nor the innate ability to de-stress.

When the adrenal system becomes weakened, the body gets sick. At this point, investigating with neuroendocrine functional diagnostics, including testing out adrenal health and supporting it can help with inflammation.

The production of low cortisol and low DHEA is most likely caused by a result of a down regulation of the HPA Axis over a long period of time, as in the case of a chronic digestive problem over years. Dealing with stress, addressing the stress, and perceiving stress differently would be a major key to healing the adrenal hormones. The way we see stress and the way we deal with it can affect everything in our system. Having the right kind of tools for stress reduction is extremely valuable.

Natural treatment options for adrenal problems would include adaptogenic herbs to decrease inflammation, nutrient support, neurotransmitter support, 5HTP, melatonin, calming herbs, phosphorylated serine, neuro steroidal support with DHEA and pregnenolone, Epsom salt baths, etc.

Adaptogenic herbs are a combination of herbal products that support the HPA Axis. Adaptogenic herbs help to moderate and turn down the volume of the stress response. These can include ashwaganda, whole basil, cordyceps, Siberian ginseng, panax ginseng, or licorice root.

Nutrient support is often necessary to respond to stressors. That requires high-potency vitamin B complex, vitamin C, magnesium, trace minerals, and zinc.

Nutritional products that are specifically created for adrenal support give good results in combination with other recommended nutrients.

Reducing inflammation with herbs is an important non-pharmaceutical treatment option because inflammation drives up cortisol levels, which can result in many negative effects including insomnia. Resolving adrenal stress will result in a better night's sleep.

Neurotransmitter support, ideally, should be considered after testing first, and those that have high levels of stress or anxiety may consider GABA, tyrosine, etc. And if there is depression, patients can consider 5HTP to support serotonin production.

Calming herbs like valerian root, passionflower, kava kava, chamomile, hops, or lemon balm can also help patients to relax and have a deeper sleep. Seriophos can be taken as a supplement for high cortisol levels and allow better sleep and less anxiety.

Neuro-steroidal support should ideally be recommended after doing functional diagnostic testing for adrenal health, and those can include DHEA and pregnenolone, which are naturally produced in the adrenals. Both DHEA and pregnenolone can be taken as drops, capsules, or tablets in the dose that would ideally be suggested after doing the adrenal testing.

Sleep is a major factor that needs to be accounted for when you're reducing stress and addressing inflammation. Our circadian rhythm directs our physical, behavioral, and mental changes. So, we must look at our sleep and the time we go to sleep. For example, making a habit of going to sleep by 11 p.m. can make a difference for your food or sugar cravings the next day. Cortisol is a glucocorticoid and is fundamental in the regulation of glucose metabolism. If cortisol is high, you'll have trouble falling asleep because glucose stores and metabolizes energy, and high energy at night can cause issues with sleep.

Being in a state of constant stress or in a fight or flight effect at night can also cause problems with falling asleep. So, sleep hygiene is one of the extremely important factors for addressing adrenal health.

Another very important treatment option that is not pharmaceutical is dietary modification. Reduce blood sugar by eating a diet that's hormone-balancing, including hormone balancing healthful oils, raw seeds, and avocado.

Maintain a diet that consists mostly of low glycemic foods, avoiding candy, juices, and processed foods. You want to add a lot of cooked vegetables, raw vegetables, low-in-sugar berries, high-quality proteins, and healthy fats. You want to eat at the same time each day, hopefully without snacks, depending on your insulin sensitivity.

Add healthful fibers, fermented foods and reduce refined sugars to a minimum.

Exercise is a great treatment option for addressing adrenal health and it's very important for many functions including lymphatic detox. Exercise for chronic patients should be more limited and not too strenuous like yoga or walking and breathing exercises. These types of exercises are sufficient for someone chronically ill.

Don't pretend that stress can just go away. Don't just sit there and wait, hoping that once you heal your stress will just go away. Deal with your stress as if it's an illness right away, so it doesn't get to a point where it becomes hard to heal yourself. You must address what's most important to your health. If Crohn's or colitis is ruining your life, there are many tools in this book, step by step, that can help you. Managing your stress should be one of them.

Stress reduction techniques can be short and should be done with good intention and will make a big difference.

Lay out new lifestyle rules. Jump out of bed early in the morning and intend for every day to be a great day starting from the morning. Meditate. Pray. Set your mood right in the morning. It makes a really big difference. After just a couple of days, you will see that it becomes easier. Your intentions and the way you set your mind can make a world of a difference. Even if you think you can't, after a few days you'll see that you'll be able to.

Learn that these Supplements Are Complementary Medicine.

This must be very clear to you. Most of functional medicine's recommended treatments are nutraceuticals.

They are not prescription medications. It's best if they are high-quality, professional nutraceuticals, but they are still not prescriptions. Working with your doctor is extremely important. Your doctor must understand that you're taking certain supplements. A professional practitioner will make sure that there are no interactions with your current medications.

That is something that you could find out from your physician, from your pharmacist, or from your functional medicine expert.

Balancing adrenals is the first and basic step in decreasing inflammation. It is hard to go further and continue with functional diagnostic testing and functional medicine without having properly balanced adrenals and decreased inflammation. It's much easier to run organic testing later and to replenish the vitamins in your body after the inflammation goes down. You will be able to absorb better, and you'll see results that much faster. So, laying the solid ground of good stable adrenal health will help you build the system without much inflammation.

Basic and General Nutraceutical Protocol for Adrenal Support:
Do not try new supplements without discussing them with your physician or healthcare practitioner first.

- Adaptogenic herbs (ex, Adaptocrine (APEX Energetics) or Adrenotone(DFH)) 1 capsule 2 to 3 times daily
- Vitamin C 1000mg with Bioflavonoids (ex, Bio Fizz (DFH) or BioFlav (OrthoMolecularProducts) 1 capsule or scoop two times daily
- Omega with Vitamin D/K/Magnesium 1 capsule two times daily

Everyone is under one form of stress or another and a certain amount of stress can be healthy and keep us productive. However, extreme stress can accumulate and start to negatively impact our health, leading to adrenal burnout. Adrenal burnout is all too common in our modern society. Some of the symptoms include: fatigue, weight gain, insomnia, irritability, and mood swings. If you suffer from any of these conditions, take the following questionnaire to identify your personal stress level.

This helpful questionnaire will give you a clue on where you are as far as adrenal health.

Adrenal Stress Profile Questionnaire

Assign each question a number between 0 and 5. You should assign values as follows:

- 0= Not true
- 3= Somewhat true
- 5= Very true

Once you have completed the questionnaire, calculate your total and locate the range you fall under in the questionnaire's scoring section.

1. I experience problems falling asleep.
2. I experience problems staying asleep.
3. I frequently experience a second wind (high energy) late at night.
4. I have energy highs and lows throughout the day.
5. I feel tired all the time.
6. I need caffeine (coffee, tea, cola, etc.) to get going in the morning.
7. I usually go to bed after 10 p.m.
8. I frequently get less than 8 hours of sleep per night.
9. I am easily fatigued.
10. Things I used to enjoy seeming like a chore lately.
11. My sex drive is lower than it used to be.
12. I suffer from depression or have recently been experiencing feelings of depression such as sadness, or loss of motivation.
13. If I skip meals I feel low energy or foggy and disoriented.
14. My ability to handle stress has decreased.
15. I find that I am easily irritated or upset.

16. I have had one or more stressful major life events (e.g., divorce, death of a loved one, job loss, new baby, new job).
17. I tend to overwork with little time for play or relaxation for extended periods of time.
18. I crave sweets.
19. I frequently skip meals or eat sporadically.
20. I am experiencing increased physical complaints such as muscle aches, headaches, or more frequent illnesses.

Scoring Your Adrenal Stress Profile:

It is important to note that this is not a diagnostic test and should not be used to diagnose any conditions. It is simply a tool to help assess your likely level of adrenal burnout.

If you scored between:

- 0-30: You are in good health.
- 30-40: You are under some stress.
- 40-50: You are a candidate for adrenal burnout.
- 50-60: You are in adrenal burnout.
- 60+: You are in severe adrenal burnout.*

**If you scored 60 or higher it is important that you take immediate steps to correct this condition before your health is adversely affected.*

If you have scored 40 or higher, you may be in adrenal burnout and will at some point experience the symptoms such as fatigue, weight issues, insomnia, irritability, and mood swings.

The role of blood sugar instability in inflammation

Blood sugar instability and insulin resistance play a role in many inflammatory conditions.

Insulin resistance happens when insulin receptors on a cell no longer respond to insulin and can result in high sugar in the blood, not yet associated with diabetes. When you eat a diet full of carbohydrates, which are broken down to sugar that's used as a fuel in the body, the amount of blood sugar can become elevated and drop too quickly. When there's a lot of glucose in the blood, the pancreas will also release a lot of insulin into the bloodstream. And when there's too much insulin in the bloodstream, the receptors get tired and stop working properly. A 2012 study was conducted at the Washington School of Medicine in St. Louis that resulted in a surprising discovery about the origin of diabetes, such as intestines. You don't have to be a diabetic to have insulin resistance. If you have insulin resistance, chances are you are not feeling great physically and emotionally and the root cause of it may be in your gut.

Blood Sugar Instability Questionnaire

Do any of the following apply to you?

1. Family history of diabetes, hypoglycemia or alcoholism
2. Calmer after meals
3. Frequent thirst
4. Night sweats (not menopausal)
5. Crave salty foods
6. Dark circles under eyes or eyes sensitive to bright light
7. More awake at night
8. Food cravings
9. Headaches
10. Irritability
11. Mood swings
12. Easily fatigued
13. Anxiety
14. Difficulty sleeping

15. Mental sluggishness
16. Eat when nervous
17. Excessive appetite for carbohydrates or sweets
18. Hungry between meals
19. Irritable before meals
20. "Shaky" if hungry
21. Lightheaded if meals are skipped
22. Low energy in the afternoon
23. Afternoon headaches
24. Crave sweets or coffee in the afternoon

If you have more than a few YES answers, chances are your blood sugar may have been unstable for quite a while and insulin resistance could be a problem.

You can talk to your healthcare practitioner about reversing this problem. The best testing for it would be checking your blood for fasting insulin, which shows up high in insulin resistance cases. You can also ask for fasting glucose testing, which shows up high in resistance cases, or SHBG (sex hormone binding globulin) which shows up low in cases of insulin resistance.

Basic healing of insulin resistance can be addressed by eating a balanced diet full of good fats and low in starchy carbohydrates (or no starchy carbohydrates at all) and occasional nutraceuticals.

Basic and General Nutraceutical Protocol for Blood Sugar Support:
Do not try new supplements without discussing them with your physician or healthcare practitioner first.

- GlucoAdopt by Douglas Labs or Glycemic Select by Moss Nutrition starting 1 capsule once daily and increasing to three times daily

- Cinnamon 1 teaspoonful once daily sprinkled on foods
- Berberine 500mg twice daily for up to 3 months. Contraindicated in medicated diabetics, pregnancy, breast-feeding, low blood pressure, and certain medications

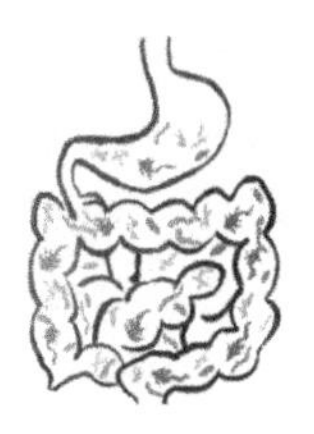

Chapter 6
FUNCTIONAL SOLUTIONS: GUT MICROBIOME IN HARMONY

"The best and most efficient pharmacy is within your own system"
– **Robert C. Peale**

Get Friendly with Your Gut Bacteria

Our beautiful microbiome has tens of trillions of microorganisms that include at least 1000 different species of known bacteria with more than 3 million genes. This is about 150 times more than human genes.

About one-third of our gut microbiome is common in most people, and the other two-thirds are unique to each of us. This makes a personal gut microbiota a personal fingerprint-like identity.

There are many autoimmune diseases, and many of them share similar triggers affecting the microbiome. When we learn what causes the immune system to break down, it will help us learn what can be done to fix it. Genetics play a role to a degree since we make our own choices about our lifestyle, where we live, our dietary and nutritional intake, etc.

The reaction of the immune system can occur in different ways. In one way, the body attacks itself, mistakenly "thinking" of its own cells as foreign during the presence of other triggers. The example here could be a virus that appears foreign to the system just because your body already is dealing with mercury as a metal toxicity.

In another example, the immune system reaction happens through cellular copying when antibodies are made for certain antigens that were produced because of opportunistic bacteria in the gut, with the final result of antibodies attacking its own tissues like the gut lining.

Another way of immune system breakdown is the development of T-cells (in the immune system). This can be affected by stress, genetics and environmental toxins. In functional medicine we look for environmental triggers, mold and toxic foods as possible root causes of immune system diseases. And the big ones to investigate would also include permeable gut (leaky gut) and dysbiosis.

Also, the immune system breakdown is dealing with xenobiotics (substances that are not natural to the body) and the total toxic burden on the body. Sometimes it's a little bit of everything that breaks the immune system.

Lots of immune system diseases need to be addressed by harmonizing gut health. I am a big believer that it all starts in the gut, and that's why I chose to specialize in gut diseases. Since I was able to address my own gut health, it became my mission to help spread the word.

Appropriate nutritional changes are effective in balancing gut flora and gut health, despite what some traditional practitioners still say. Sometimes it's advantageous to add antimicrobials, digestive enzymes, prebiotics, probiotics, herbals and adrenal supplements to balance the gut microbiota even better.

Some functional medicine specialists use different sequences of the 4-R approach to improve gut health, and I find this sequence to be most effective in my practice.

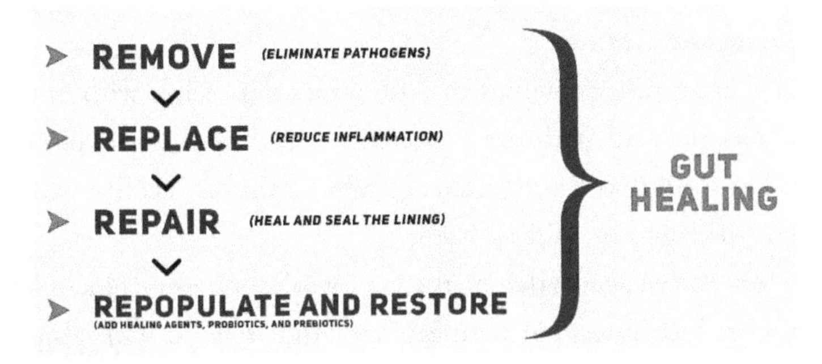

Remove:

Through correct stool testing it would be important to eliminate pathogenic viruses, fungi, bacteria, and parasites. There are options to get rid of those using longer therapy with herbals. These may include caprylic acid, sweet wormwood, grapefruit extract, berberine, and others.

Replace:

Using digestive enzymes in the cases of inflamed gut is often very helpful. Those individuals who are under stress and experiencing inflammation often do not secrete enough enzyme called protease, not enough acid and can develop allergies, colitis, autoimmune diseases, and more.

Repair:

The repair step needs to be started at the right time. The right time to repair during the functional medicine program is after the adrenals are supported, which decreases inflammation, and after pathogens (unfriendly gut visitors) are cleared. If you start a healing and repairing agent too soon, like L-glutamine, for example, you can often cause an irritable gut reaction, but not always. Some patients benefit from L-glutamines support right away. Glutamine is very important for colonocytes of the large intestine and is responsible for healthy gut cells. It's used to prevent permeable, or leaky, gut.

Repopulate and Restore:

Choosing appropriate prebiotics and probiotics helps with nutrient assimilation, prevents pathogenic bacterial overgrowth, and replaces the bacteria lost to antibiotic use (often taken by Crohn's and colitis patients), bad diet, stress, and the disease itself.

There are other agents that do the same work as N-acetyl glucosamine, known to reduce intestinal permeability. And it helps with abnormal T-cell growth, diverting the attack on the body. Sometimes L-glutamine is used with N-acetyl glucosamine in combination with agents that oppose the production of gut mucus, including slippery elm, marshmallow, chamomile, cat's claw, okra, and DGL. They also act as soothing and coating agents to comfort the inflamed gut.

If the immune system is overloaded with toxins, stress, toxic foods, and even toxic thoughts, the expected result would be destruction. Getting all these back in shape takes time and patience.

The microflora in the lumen of patients with IBDs is characterized by decreased commensal bacterial load, especially Bacteroidetes and Firmicutes. Newer genetic research utilizes different, very specific laboratory testing using a panel that includes genetic and immunological markers. With this new technology, there's less room for human error and more room for a correct bug identification. Also, PCR testing is now used in gut microbiology, including PCR stool testing for testing commensal bacteria, parasites, gut infection, and inflammatory markers. The identification couldn't be as precise before as it is today. And the role of probiotics becomes even more important now that we will be able to manipulate GI flora better.

Examples of common intestinal health markers found on PCR stool diagnostics:

- Secretory IgA, marker for immune system
- Anti-gliadin IgA, marker for gluten sensitivity
- Calprotectin, marker of the gut inflammation, usually significantly higher in IBD patients
- Zonulin, marker for leaky gut or intestinal permeability
- Steatocrit, marker for fat absorption
- Elastase-1, marker for digestive activity

Looking into the amounts of the bacteria present in your stool and ruling out pathogenic growth can become an extremely important step in gut healing. Only after you are done removing can you start replacing, inoculating, and repairing.

Probiotics

When our immune system is working effectively, "friendly" bacteria maintain balance and helps get rid of harmful pathogens. In contrast, an imbalance may result from bacterial overgrowth of harmful pathogens and present symptoms such diarrhea, pain, bloating, and others. That's where probiotics come in to replenish good bacterial storage. Currently, probiotics are available in different forms including capsules, powders, or tablets, and as dietary supplements or probiotic-labeled foods like yogurt, fermented soy, fermented miso, fermented and unfermented milk, fermented tempeh, kombucha, and others.

Although the mechanism of action of probiotics isn't completely understood, probiotics can stimulate lymphocyte and macrophage activity as well as cytokine production, and therefore work as immunomodulators that can increase IgA (secretory immune globulin A) in the intestine, improving the immune system's response. Bifidobacterium and Lactobacillus are the two genera of bacteria most commonly found in probiotic supplements. They are also naturally occurring in your gut. There have been some studies linking the beneficial use of certain strains of Lactobacillus, like L. salivarius, L. plantarum, and L. rhamnosus GG, although those studies had poor data.

There is more evidence now suggesting that probiotics may help Crohn's or ulcerative colitis patients to maintain remission. Some studies show that probiotics can be helpful for preventing and treating pouchitis (which can occur after removing the colon). Probiotic use is a great new way to balance microflora. Its safety has been shown consistently, except in some cases of immunocompromised patients who may experience worsening of their condition.

Some other evidence against using probiotics like S. Boulardii in Crohn's disease is based on speculation of possible fungal overgrowth.

The history of probiotic use in Crohn's disease goes back to the early twentieth century, when a product called Metaflor (E.coli Nissle) was researched by a German physician investigating fecal flora of soldiers fighting in the war, as well as what product can help and what efficacy to expect. The discovery of this strand of E.coli as an effective probiotic for bowel disease was made in the early 20th century by Dr. Nissle.

Probiotics are effective in improving the microbiota of the gut. Currently, gut microbiota is considerably studied and believed to affect many functions of the body, including neutralizing toxins, communicating and re-training the immune system, balancing the microflora of the gut, preventing the growth of pathogenic organisms, and producing vitamins including vitamin K and biotin and short chain fatty acids

Feeding the Good Bacteria: Foods for Healthy Gut and Healthy Gut Microbiome

Cruciferous Vegetables like Cauliflower, Kale, Broccoli and Collard Greens:
The powerful compound called sulforaphane is the staple of the cruciferous foods listed above. Sulforaphane is a sulfur-containing compound that reverses aging, stops inflammation, kills cancer, protects the brain, and is even advantageous in cardiovascular disease. These vegetables must be prepared and eaten appropriately to maximize the bioavailability of sulforaphane. Broccoli sprouts have much more sulforaphane than all the other cruciferous vegetables combined.

Best way to cook cruciferous foods for your gut: chop them first and then let them sit for 20-30 minutes. Do not use very high temperatures, to avoid destroying the beneficial effects. It's best to steam or stir-fry them to keep most nutrients.

Freshly Ground Flax Seed or Freshly Ground Chia Seed:
These are high in fiber and are insoluble (due to bulkiness), which improves bowel movements, helps improve the gut microbiome, and binds and helps to remove toxins. They are rich in omega fatty acids that also coat the gut lining and help with easier transport of toxins and stool out of the gut. Flax seeds contain lignans, which are studied as protection against breast, colon, and prostate cancers, hormone imbalance, and heart disease.

Bone Broth:
One of the best foods for gut health! Bone broth is a wonderful source of collagen, a protein that the intestinal lining depends on. Collagen has been researched for improvements in IBS and IBD (Crohn's and colitis)

and permeable gut. Some research shows that IBD patients naturally produce less collagen in their gut.

When collagen intakes are optimized, it can balance mucus membranes, make GI tissues stronger, and help close tight junctions (in cases of leaky gut). As a result, the undigested food particles and other substances won't leak into the system. When collagen is broken down it forms a gelatin substance. Adding bone broth can even help cases with food intolerance to dairy and gluten. It contains glycine, proline, and glutamine. All these amino acids are great for gut healing and bacterial balance.

Jerusalem Artichoke:

This is a prebiotic food that has indigestible fibers, and when traveling into your small intestine it can feed good bacteria in the microbiome-rich colon. This isn't a regular artichoke. It looks more like a ginger root. Jerusalem artichoke contains a third of the fiber by weight, and it feeds a healthy microbiome. Added to soups or salads, it provides a great prebiotic food for good gut flora.

Garlic:

Garlic is known for its anti-fungal properties. Very often overgrowth of candida is a major cause of symptoms like gas, constipation, bloating, rosacea, and acne. Garlic is also a great prebiotic, which feeds good bacteria and creates a great microbiome.

Sauerkraut, Pickled, Fermented Foods, and Kimchi:

The process of fermentation creates a powerhouse of good gut bacteria and gives a chance for the gut to balance the flora without even probiotic supplements. Using fermented foods like sauerkraut, kimchi, and pickled veggies will support gut microbiome and improve the immune system function.

Vegetables as Natural Fiber:

Veggies are super rich in prebiotics and increasing fiber rich foods will increase the ability to absorb probiotics. Foods like onions, asparagus, chicory root, dandelion greens, and even plantains are wonderful prebiotic sources for a great microbiome.

Celery Juice:

This very effective, alkaline juice made from fresh organic celery will heal the gut, and the natural minerals found in this juice will balance out the gut microbiome. Organic celery juice helps digestion, hormones, immune health, and brain health. It also has luteolin, which decreases inflammation. With added ginger and lemon, you can create a powerful microbiome supporting drink.

Apple Cider Vinegar:

ACV seems to be very well tolerated and helps with digestion. It can also help build a stronger microbiome.

Leaky Gut (Intestinal Permeability)

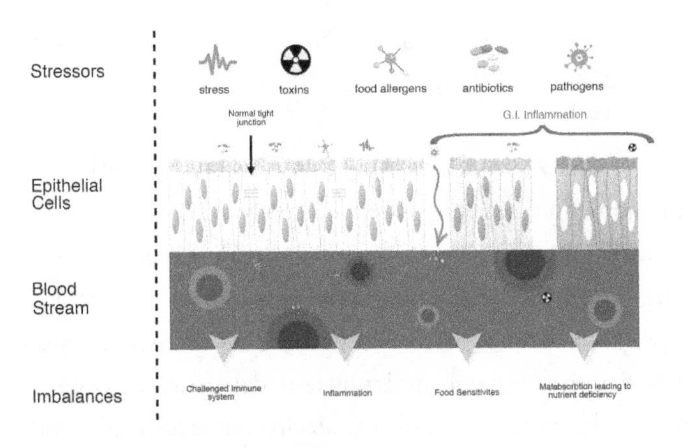

Leaky gut is the result of the chronic inflammatory attacks on the gut lining by different triggers like gluten, chemicals, allergens, toxins, etc. resulting in intestinal permeability. An easy way to describe this phenomenon would be to compare the intestinal tissue to a porous strainer which we need to heal and seal. It's almost like patching up a piece of clothing that has holes in it.

It is very important to address leaky gut because if the lining is repaired, it's easier to address gut infections, candida, food allergies, sensitivities, and more.

Basic and General Nutraceutical Protocol for Leaky Gut:

Do not try new supplements without discussing them with your physician or healthcare practitioner first.

- L-glutamine powder up to 5 grams three times daily (I prefer Ortho Molecular Products, Design for Health and Pure Encapsulations) can be used as a combination product with NAC, N-Acetyl-D-Glucosamine and Lactoferrin
- Digestive Enzymes 1 capsule three times daily before meals
- Milk Thistle 2 capsules twice daily
- Liposomal Glutathione 100mg once daily or NAC up to 1500mg once daily

SIBO (Small Intestinal Bacterial Overgrowth)

This phenomenon happens when normally present bacteria overgrow in the small intestine, where it's not normally meant to be present in such large quantities. As a result, the involvement of bacteria there is associated with damage to the lining or mucosal barrier, causing leaky gut and vitamin, mineral, and nutrient deficiencies. More and more uncomfortable gas is produced. Fat absorption is affected, food allergies and sensitivities develop, immune system reactions develop, and even cognitive symptoms can result.

There's a lot of research linking SIBO to IBDs. There are more studies connecting it to Crohn's than colitis. The numbers in the studies vary, but at least 25% of Crohn's disease patients are associated with SIBO. Some studies report a 59% remission rate after treatment with an antibiotic-like medication named Rifaximin. It's a unique drug in a class of its own and it's used for SIBO.

The reason I chose to highlight SIBO as a part of the microbiome chapter versus the root causes chapter is because it is a Small Intestinal Bacterial Overgrowth that is associated with microbiome issues.

When there's damage to the gut lining, the bacteria will interfere with the way we digest and absorb food. That will create numerous problems, including malabsorption of B12 and iron, causing anemia and fatigue.

It can lead to poor absorption of fats, leading to malabsorption of vitamins A and D and cause fatty, leaky stools. The food particles are not well digested, and it causes the body to have an autoimmune reaction, food allergies, intolerance, and food sensitivities.

Bacteria can enter the bloodstream. As a result, the immune system reacts to bacteria and endotoxins (a toxin released when a bacterial cell wall disintegrates), which can cause chronic fatigue and irritate the liver.

There's a lot of gas produced by bacteria, and SIBO patients have uncomfortable bloating, gas, belching, gut pain, diarrhea, or constipation.

In worst cases, the overgrowth of the bacteria in the small intestine can excrete acids that, in high amounts, can lead to cognitive and neurological symptoms like brain fog, depression, loss of concentration, and more.

Now there are different tests available on the market to investigate SIBO further. Most of them used today are breath tests. Breath tests will measure methane and hydrogen produced by bacteria in the small intestine that is diffused into the blood and then the lungs. Patients first get prepped with a special two-day diet. The prep diet excludes most carbohydrates and they are limited to mostly animal proteins and water, allowing for a clear reaction to the sugary drink. Then they drink a sugar or glucose liquid to measure the results. Those gases are not produced by us, but by the bacteria. They will measure out the transit time of two or three hours and will compare it to a baseline.

Treating SIBO is very tricky even if you find the most advanced gastroenterologist. There are options with antibiotics, herbal antimicrobials, and diet, as well as an elemental diet that can be homemade, but very difficult to comply with. Most of my clients' report being very hungry during this two-week elemental diet. It is very important to use stress reduction in SIBO cases since stress makes it so much worse. Stay very patient, drink herbal teas, be consistent with the diet, and avoid sugars at all costs.

Pharmacologic Treatment Includes:

Do not try new medications without discussing them with your physician or healthcare practitioner first.

- Rifaxamin 1,200 to 1,600 mg once daily (dose depends on whether it's methane or hydrogen producing SIBO) and is sometimes combined with metronidazole or neomycin.

Basic and General Nutraceutical Protocol for SIBO:

Do not try new supplements without discussing them with your physician or healthcare practitioner first.

- Candicid Forte 2 capsules three times daily
- Oil of Oregano 1-2 capsules three times daily, depending on tolerability

- In cases of methane producing SIBO, adding a garlic supplement is also recommended

Fecal Transplants:

FMT (Fecal Microbiota Transplantation) is a new therapeutic procedure that restores intestinal microbiota by using a healthy subject's material. Recurrent infections of Clostridium difficile were successfully treated by FMT in 83–92% of patients. There's more data coming out and this therapeutic approach seems very promising to stabilize the GI microbiota.

Currently only patients with C. Difficile have FDA approval to receive fecal transplants. This is only done through reputable, experienced doctors. If more quality data comes to the surface from FMT case studies, there's a chance that the FDA will approve it for other chronic gut situations.

Parasitic Infections.

While we don't think of parasitic infections as a problem in developed counties, in functional medicine exploring the gut flora and looking for possible parasites is a must. Some parasites can be found in small quantities that do not cause harm to the host, while others can be that initial trigger, that root cause which tipped off the illness.

Basic and General Nutraceutical Protocol for Parasite Cleanse:

Do not try new supplements without discussing them with your physician or healthcare practitioner first.

- Artemisia 2 capsules two to three times daily
- Oil of oregano 1 capsule one to three times daily
- Combo Herbal Anti Parasitic Supplement GI Microb-X (DFH) or Tricycline (Allergy Research Group) 1 capsule two to three times daily

Candida

Fungal infections can be very serious and even life threatening for immunocompromised people. Having fungal microbiota, dysbiosis or candida overgrowth showing in stool was found to play a possible role as root cause for IBD. A study published in the *Gut Journal* in June of 2017 suggests that fungal growth as well as pathogenic bacteria overgrowth has an effect on IBDs. There are pharmacological treatments for fecal fungal overgrowth, including nystatin, which is a prescription medicine, and natural medicines as well.

Basic and General Nutraceutical Protocol for Candida:

Do not try new supplements without discussing them with your physician or healthcare practitioner first.

- Candicid Forte 2 capsules three times daily
- Oil of Oregano 1–2 capsules three times daily, depending on tolerability
- Purified Colloidal Silver 15 ppm once daily

The key to remember with these powerful, natural antimicrobials is that they may also deplete the flora of good bacteria, so it's very important to colonize your gut afterwards with a great probiotic.

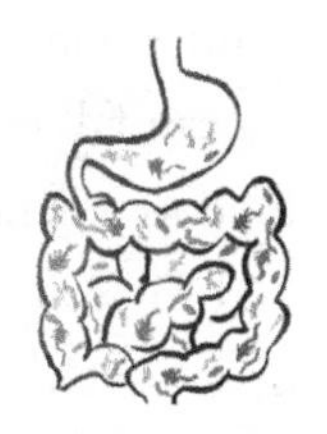

Chapter 7
FUNCTIONAL SOLUTIONS: FEAR FOOD NO MORE, PEACEFUL DIGESTION

"We gain strength, and courage, and confidence by each experience in which we really stop to look fear in the face.
– Eleanor Roosevelt

Fear No More

Before you read this chapter, I want to remind you that I have never been trained in psychology or the psychology of eating. Everything I am suggesting here is from my own personal and clinical experience.

Many digestive sufferers start seeing food as an enemy, and you can't blame them. When you constantly have pain after eating, when you constantly have unbearable gas after eating, you will start getting uncomfortable.

Anxiety about food comes from reasonable pain, overload of information, or from despair. As functional medicine specialists, we help you heal the physical body, so you can fall in love with food again.

How can we re-focus from food as an enemy to food as a friend? For some it can be a slow process and for others it can be smooth sailing. Those that often get help from a psychotherapist or hypnotherapist for severe emotional attachments to food can do much better with a functional medicine approach. Just think about addressing a big problem from both ends and you'll realize that getting to your goal is easier and faster than you thought.

Methods that clean and clear out your subconscious can be done for any kind of fear at any point in the treatment. These could be EFT (emotional freedom technique exercises), hypnotherapy sessions, or deep meditation.

And if you want a methodological approach to stop fearing foods, this is what worked for many of my clients:

Confront your fears.

You must realize that this is not an actual fear of food; it is the fear of pain after eating, or other possible negative effects that you are expecting. In the back of your mind, you know it is not the food.

Start writing down what really makes you fear your foods and what is the worst thing that could happen if you eat it. For most Crohn's/colitis/digestive patients it is a very real pain. But others are so exhausted from the illness that they now develop an unreasonable fear. The examples of those could be: "I'll eat this piece of meat and will have pain so bad that my intestines will rupture, and I will die." This is a real fear from a real patient. But maybe the fear isn't that real—maybe it has become unreasonable—and seeing it in your journal can be a therapeutic and very important exercise.

Make a quiet mealtime a priority.

Get rid of your phone, Facebook groups, TV or your computer. Just sit down and eat. Pray or set an intention first. And then eat. Decorate your plate—make a smiley face on your plate! Even if it's a mashed soup, you can add two blueberries on top like eyes and a cooked carrot as a mouth. Play with it, and then chew very slowly. Get a taste of the food, breathe slowly, and swallow with the intention to digest well. This is a mindful process that may take a while to perfect, but it's so worth it. It's best if you journal what you eat and how you feel afterwards.

Respecting and loving your body and therefore choosing foods that benefit it.

Re-train yourself from saying, "I can't have gluten and it sucks," to, "I am choosing to avoid gluten because it's best for my body right now." Or instead of, "I'll avoid chocolate because I will get migraines, but it stinks," you now say, "I love my body enough that I'm avoiding chocolate to feel awesome."

After reading this book you'll learn that quality foods are best for digestive disease. Quality foods contain no additives, no artificial colors, no trans fats, no extra sugars, etc. You are what you eat, and you eat well now. Go for organic, clean, non-GMO brands. Choose raw nuts and seeds, since roasting can change fat composition and reduce vitamin E content. If you love sweets you can add a small amount of maple syrup or raw honey to the nuts and seeds. Choose whole foods as your staples, such as quality meats, vegetables, and good oils.

Do not buy foods that you're trying to avoid. It works! When you know that chocolate is in the pantry, you will go and grab it over and over. When you are shopping in the supermarket and you get stuck next to the potato chip section, giving yourself an excuse like, "it's just for the kids," stop. The kids don't need it either—you know it.

Learn to trust yourself again and trust your gut.

Sit down before eating, breathe, and ask your intuition what advice it would give you, what food would it recommend to you. If you indulge, accept it with love and appreciation for yourself, with a strong intention to avoid it the next time.

Helping the digestion process will help the pain and therefore help with the fear of food.

Using prayers before meals doesn't need to be religion-related, if you are not into it, but just setting intent for digestion before eating will play a positive role. Digestive enzymes can be used for occasional indigestion or pain after eating to help the inflamed system digest better.

Starting with a spoon of apple cider vinegar (ACV) can help in cases of low gastric acid. When you are about to start eating, take some apple cider vinegar (ACV) to stimulate gastric acid production. Also, take 3 deep breaths right before eating to make the pH even more beneficial for digestion. This will help digestion and assimilation of nutrients go so much smoother.

Another problem that I see with some patients is the fear of staying with the same practitioner. Doctor-hopping can get overwhelming. You think that the next doctor or the next test will get you the results you want without having to put in the work and become friends with food again.

Mindful Eating

This is a term I learned not too long ago and boy, am I happy I learned about it. We have not been treating the eating process with respect! We never learned the entire biochemical, psychological, and emotional aspects of the eating process. It is super complex, from the first smell and bite of food to swallowing, digesting, assimilating, and excreting. The process is so smart and advanced, and we do not use it to our advantage. There can be so much improvement if there's a mindful approach to our eating habits.

A large percentage of us will eat at work, while continuing our jobs, looking at our computer screens, and talking on the phone at the same time. This will decrease the gastric acid secretions, enzymatic production, and digestive functions, which can result in fewer nutrients absorbed, more food eaten, with more calories and less nutrient content.

There's something very scientific about praying before meals, sitting down for dinner with an entire family for hours, eating, and having family conversations. No TV, no phones, and no computers. If you have digestive problems, it is also in your hands to teach your children how to avoid having the same problems. And simply, eating together as a family in the evening with no gadgets can help digestion.

As functional medicine practitioners we are all about eating right. But it doesn't only mean the right kind of foods. It also means having enough gastric acid when you start chewing, as well as enough digestive enzymes secreted by the pancreas to digest the meal and enough bile acids to do the excretion part of the digestive process. All those must be functioning properly and if you add healthy foods to that healthy mind picture now we have a successful digestive process.

Digestive organs involved in our body are very complex. The colon itself is responsible for many functions. Digestive system functions are directly responsible for our good health. That's if we are being good to ourselves.

The digestive system is affected by our emotions. Learning more about emotions and how they connect to certain points of the body and learning how to release the blocks can benefit and even have an analgesic effect for the digestive system.

The malfunction of our beautifully designed body usually starts because we do something inappropriate to it, and it's not just physical but also emotional: poor diet, stress, anxiety and chemicals in our environment can all be the cause for this malfunction. And that's how digestive system diseases start.

My acupuncturist once told me that in Eastern medicine people love with their liver not with their heart. This means that the liver is so important in the digestive process that it becomes the main organ. So, we should take care of it. Very sensitive people have more digestive problems for a reason. The liver reacts instantly to stress, causing the gall bladder to alter the production of bile. And that starts the vicious cycle of abdominal distress.

The digestive system is like a fine instrument. If you mistreat your body, it will remind you of it in the most inappropriate time. So, learn to respect and nourish your inside! This system is the engine of our health. This is where you get all the nutrition for every cell in your body. The immune system depends on it as well.

When the digestive system is inflamed, like in IBD cases, or you are constipated or irritated, it simply cannot do its job and will cause health problems. But the good news is, we can actually do something natural to repair and retain good digestive health.

Start listening to your body and pay close attention to it. If the liver doesn't tolerate certain foods, try to avoid them. You will know when you get abdominal cramps (primarily on the right side), nausea, indigestion, etc.

If you slip up and drink a can of soda, it's not just one innocent drink. It's 10 teaspoonfuls of sugar in your body, which turns into a vicious cycle of your body craving even more sugar. High sugar intake has been associated with possible causes of IBDs. For many IBD patients the inability to digest the foods appropriately can cause flatulence, especially after sugar intake.

Ideally, the human body should be able to fight off some viruses and infections without the use of antibiotics, and a healthy liver should be able to filter out most toxins and chemicals from your body. With Crohn's patients, it becomes complicated because our immune system is often over-active, and it needs help to stay in balance. We must always be on guard. Our digestive system is not going to be very forgiving! If you want to stay symptom-free, you will need to be very strict with yourself, at least in the beginning No cheating with your diet! And get enough rest!

Every human system is unique, and I wish that was recognized more by doctors. I realized that one person might do very well with one product while someone else may not tolerate it at all. For example, I tried one new product extracted from hops. It had many great supportive studies. It was really promising on paper as natural cancer prevention and much more. Many people loved this product and improved their sleep and health using it. But I just got horrible migraines while taking it.

I am a lucky Crohn's patient, in a sense, since I can better understand medicine because I am a pharmacist. Even though I am a pharmacist, I try to lean toward more natural healing to repair the digestive system, because a lot of times the natural solution is the way to minimize side effects. And mindful eating can be that missing puzzle piece for great digestion.

I still think that traditional medicine is indispensable in many ways, but there is so much room for complementary style medicine to address most aspects of your health, and mindful eating needs to be a part of the plan. Be grateful if your symptoms are under control, and stick to healthy habits and a healthy diet. Because, for IBD patients, if you slip up just a little, you will pay a lot later. Let's treat our digestive system with respect, face those fears, and start the healing process with excitement and trust that you will heal!

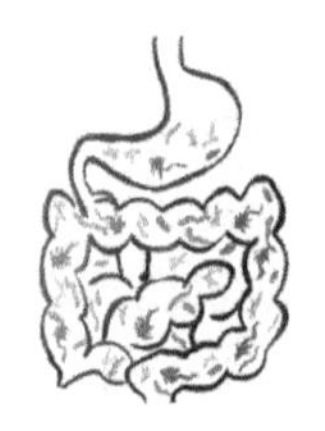

Chapter 8
FUNCTIONAL SOLUTIONS: ANTI-INFLAMMATORY DIET

"Let food be thy medicine and medicine be thy food."
– **Hippocrates**

Diet Works?

If you've been recently diagnosed or have had IBD for a while, you may have realized that eating right is a big part of correcting the inflammation. When I was diagnosed, my gastroenterologist told me I should be able to eat whatever I want and feel okay. That of course required me to be on multiple medications. Medications are not without side effects. And what if I chose to eat the foods that did not inflame my gut? That option wasn't discussed with my doctor. I hope many things have changed since 2003, but I know that some doctors are still not advocating for an anti-inflammatory dietary approach.

Although many patients still take the option of eating whatever they want and staying on medications, that was not an option for me for many reasons. First, as a pharmacist, I knew every side effect there was, and just knowing them all can make you sick to your stomach. And like many of my clients and other Crohn's/colitis patients I was very sensitive to drugs. I felt super exhausted by them. I couldn't live my life being that tired.

As a major part of functional medicine, the use of an anti-inflammatory or healing diet contributes to significant changes in the inflammatory process. We incorporate the healing diet as a first, basic, and very important step to healing. That is the step where you will contribute most of the efforts on your own and with that you can bring fun and enthusiasm to your healing journey.

For some, starting with an elimination diet is a great first choice. The elimination diet process can be fun if you start it with a clear intention to learn more about your body, your temple. During an elimination diet process, you remove major food allergens (eight foods account for about 90 percent of all food-allergy reactions) such as: milk, eggs, peanuts, nuts, gluten/wheat, soy, fish, and shellfish. Then you add foods back in slowly one by one. If you think of an elimination diet as a difficult process, you may skip that step for the meantime, because stressing out is the last thing you want when trying to heal. Some choose to do a food intolerance test to know what they can or cannot eat. And ideally you want to start a food/mood/bowel movement diary for more clarity. It serves very well if you are working with a functional medicine guide.

If you are ready to start a simpler version, go for the eliminating foods process by taking out foods like gluten, dairy, and soy. There's scientific data supporting coexistence of celiac presence in some Crohn's patients, as well as positive changes from a low-FODMAP diet in inflammatory bowel diseases. FODMAP are fermentable carbohydrates that may aggravate the stomach lining in those prone to food sensitivities. Those foods include milk, yogurt, soft cheese, figs, mangoes, blackberries, agave nectar, wheat, rye, legumes, some sweeteners, etc. And numerous studies support that a gluten-free diet can improve clinical symptoms in patients with IBD.

Commit to do it for an entire four weeks and pay attention to the way you feel and to your symptoms. I strongly suggest starting a food diary. And be completely honest with it—it's your health, after all. It may become a valuable tool to fix your gut.

FOOD DIARY WEEK OF ______________

	SUN	MON	TUE	WED	THU	FRI	SAT
BREAKFAST Time:_______ Effect on bowel movement							
SNACK Time:_______ Effect on bowel movement							
LUNCH Time:_______ Effect on bowel movement							
SNACK Time:_______ Effect on bowel movement							
DINNER Time:_______ Effect on bowel movement							
SNACK Time:_______ Effect on bowel movement							

If you notice that the same food makes you react, simply avoid it for four weeks then re-start to see how you are feeling. Getting into more complex elimination diet details during a more detailed and longer GI healing program is always an option in functional medicine. This is only a four week quick start.

Fluid Intake:

Pay attention to how much water you are drinking. Good hydration will yield natural detoxification benefits. Get into the habit of drinking water with a little bit of essence in it—like lemon or lime.

Drinking good quality water will not only hydrate your body, but it will also help your body clear out unwanted toxins. You should drink at least half ounce of water per pound of your body weight. For example, someone who weighs 120 pounds should drink at least 60 ounces of water. That's around 2 liters of water.

Our body sends a signal when we are thirsty and often we misinterpret this signal as being hungry. If you have chosen to take steps to improve your gut—under doctor's supervisions of course—your homework would be to keep your clean, pure water next to you all the time.

Make sure you are drinking from glass or stainless-steel containers (aluminum free preferred). Plastic bottles are associated with leaking estrogen-like compounds into the water. Also, get into the habit of drinking a spoonful of ACV (apple cider vinegar) mixed with tiny bit of water just before every large meal to help you with acid and enzyme production for better digestion.

Fiber Intake:

Make sure that you are consuming plenty of natural fiber and prebiotics daily. Why? Fiber is not just great for better stool formation, but it also helps get rid of toxins better. You don't want to store toxins in a system that's already inflamed, so let's start with tiny amounts of fiber/prebiotics and build it up in small quantities to avoid uncomfortable gas formation.

And what foods have those prebiotics?

First, start with raw greens, raw dandelion greens, raw leeks, raw garlic, chia seeds, raw onion, and asparagus. Ideally you want to make sure there's at least 5 grams of prebiotic fiber in your daily diet. For example, you would need about 120 grams (3/4 lbs.) of raw asparagus daily or 25 grams (1 ounce) of raw dandelion greens a day. If calculating your fiber intake is way too complex on a busy day, just remember, eating at least 3 large portions of raw greens and other raw colorful veggies daily would do the trick.

Some of you are familiar with the fact that your healthy and balanced gut flora (gut microbiota) is very important for overall health. We are talking about your gastrointestinal flora now. Look at your tongue in the mirror. Is your tongue nice and pink? Or does it have a white or grey film covering it?

If you're like many people, unfortunately, your tongue isn't a perfect pink color. Having white film on your tongue often indicates candida overgrowth or bacterial overgrowth and you want to take care of that. How about clearing it up? Your tongue says a lot about your gastrointestinal health. In Eastern medicine the tongue is like a map for diagnosing. Working on balancing the flora in your gut can make tremendous changes in the way you feel, how well you absorb nutrients, and much more. And as a result, your entire body, not just your gut, will benefit from having a healthier immune system. And often, natural treatments for clearing up the tongue include probiotic phages, like ProBiophage DF from Designs For Health, herbal anti-microbials like berberine, potent probiotics, soil-based probiotics and more.

Probiotics as part of the dietary change:

Probiotics play a tremendous role in balancing your gut microflora. Probiotics are effective in improving the microbiota of the gut. Currently, gut microbiota is considerably studied and believed to affect many functions of the body, including neutralizing toxins, communicating and re-training the immune system, preventing the growth of pathogenic organisms, balancing the microflora of the gut, and producing vitamins, including vitamin K, biotin, and short chain fatty acids. Probiotics are not to be confused with prebiotics. Probiotics are beneficial bacteria that can improve gut-related symptoms and promote better overall health, while prebiotics are the food that feeds the probiotics (good bacteria) so they can grow and do their job efficiently.

Evaluating probiotics in clinical management of Crohn's and colitis should really be a priority. Even fecal transplants are now successfully used to improve gut flora because they recolonize the gut with naturally occurring probiotics.

As far as different blends of probiotics, which one is the one for you? With so many different brands out there, it's difficult to decide what probiotic to choose. Ideally you want to choose a blend that's a mix of Bifido and Lactobacillus, or potent Megaspores show great benefit. They need to be evaluated with your health care professional. You may want to avoid the ingredient S. thermophilus, since many Crohn's and colitis patients report being more irritated with this ingredient. The better way to choose your probiotic is with a good PCR technology functional stool analysis that will allow you to see what your commensal bacteria is like.

What can we use for balancing gut flora besides probiotic supplements?

Fermented foods as probiotic foods. It would be very beneficial to start adding cultured and fermented foods. Why? Because it's a great way, if not the best way, to absorb natural probiotics. According to numerous studies, probiotics from foods are very beneficial for gut health and our microbiome.

Probiotic foods improve immune system function and skin appearance, help in reducing allergies, help Crohn's and colitis patients, and much more.

So, what other foods have natural probiotics?

- Sour pickles
- Organic miso soups—make sure there's no gluten

- Cultured coconut kefir or coconut milk
- Kombucha
- Sauerkraut

You can even culture or ferment your own veggies or other foods. It's an art in and of its own. And I haven't mastered it yet, but I know gut health experts that use fermented foods as a staple of their programs. There are terrific benefits to eating fermented foods because they are full of naturally-occurring probiotics that are easier to digest and absorb.

What else can I do to tame my gut inflammation?

Starting to eliminate artificial sweeteners and additives and limiting sugar intake will not only help you to detox better, but also reduce candida burden, help the gut flora, improve metabolism, and so much more. Eliminating artificial additives can be as simple as not buying any products with the word "artificial" in their ingredients.

Also, too many ingredients and "chemical"-sounding ingredients can be a red flag that something is not healthy. With sugar content, ideally if your gut is not in great shape, you want to maintain a maximum of 25 grams of sugar from all your foods daily for the next 10 weeks. This will help with yeast related problems if you have them, or it will help prevent them if you tend to have yeast. Reducing sugar intake will also retrain your brain and you will have fewer sugar cravings after just 23 days (roughly three weeks).

Should I stop eating meat to improve my Crohn's/colitis?

Semi-Vegetarian Diet (SVD) and Reducing Animal Protein

A recent prospective two-year clinical study considered Crohn's disease patients who achieved remission on a semi-vegetarian diet as a preventative measure. Those patients were in high risk group for relapse of Crohn's.

This trial compared Crohn's disease patients who ate an omnivorous diet (meat-based group) to those with a semi-vegetarian diet. The results were that 94% of patients on a semi-vegetarian diet (compared to 33% of those who ate meat predominately) achieved a remission rate (where no symptoms of Crohn's disease occurred). And C-reactive protein (a marker for inflammation) was normal in more than half of the patients who were on a semi-vegetarian diet. So as a conclusion of this study, SVD was highly effective in preventing relapse in CD.

What does SVD consists of? Mostly plant foods, dairy products (which you will be avoiding for now), eggs, and occasional (possibly once a week) chicken, fish, and red meat.

Animal Protein and IBDs

This was a large French study that evaluated diet and the role of dietary macronutrients in the etiology of inflammatory bowel disease. They evaluated women, aged 40–65 years, with no disease at the beginning of the study. Among 67,581 participants, they validated 77 incident IBD cases. High total protein intake, specifically animal protein, was associated with a much higher risk of IBD, for total and animal protein. Among sources of animal protein, high consumption of meat or fish, but not of eggs or dairy products was associated with IBD risk.

As a conclusion of this study: high protein intake is associated with an increased risk of incident IBD in French middle-aged women.

Looking at this study, it's still not transparent whether participants had veggies with their protein, and some aspects are still unknown, but from the clinical experience in functional medicine it seems that inflamed patients seemed to do well on a semi-vegetarian diet, including bone broth for a short detox period.

What type of diet would be recommended?

When I work with my IBD clients it's never one diet fits all. But what seemed to work for many and myself was to stay mostly low-carb paleo with occasional semi-vegetarian cleanses that combine soups and smoothies during season changes, after holidays, or simply when my body signals me it's time for a cleanse.

Adding omega rich foods into the diet is another anti-inflammatory kick start. Studies suggest that new fish oil supplementation that limits the side effects of older fish oil therapy shows promise as an adjunctive treatment for Crohn's disease. Many new studies support omega rich foods for gut healing.

Ingredient combinations that should be avoided are carrageenan-containing products since this can irritate the GI tract. For others it can be nuts and seeds that are irritating to the gut lining, especially during flares, although they contain a lot of nutrition and can be considered healing foods. Using seeds and certain nuts in a nut or seed butter form can be a good option to try. Other ingredients to avoid would be sorbitol, mannitol, maltitol, and xylitol, which are sugar alcohols. They have been studied and proven to be poorly absorbed in the small intestine, consequently entering the colon, where they are subject to anaerobic fermentation and therefore make you bloated, gassy and uncomfortable.

In my recent interview on the *Low Carb Paleo Show* I mentioned that a low carb paleo diet will suppress candida, support the gut with a sufficient amount of amino acids, support adrenal//hormonal health, and will have an anti-inflammatory effect.

Smoothies:

And I'm not talking about sweet fruit smoothies. I mean nutrient dense veggie/berry smoothies. Those will be healing for your gut. How important are those smoothies? Think about your inflamed or leaky gut for a moment. It's hard to absorb nutrients for those with Crohn's and colitis. Pain is associated with every bite in many patients. So why not make it easy and smart for your gut to digest and absorb that nutrition?

My Green Smoothie Recipe:

- Pack of Baby Spinach
- 1/2 of a Banana (only if there's no dysbiosis, SIBO or candida present)
- Half a pack of frozen blueberries
- 1–2 dates (only if there's no dysbiosis, SIBO or candida)
- 3 tablespoons raw pumpkin seeds
- Use unsweetened dairy-free milk of your choice (coconut, almond, cashew, or hemp), add 1 scoop of collagen powder at the end

I use a Vitamix to mix my smoothies and try having them daily. Take notes, keep your food diary, and listen to your gut when you are about to eat something you should not.

So, what anti-inflammatory foods can balance and heal hormones?

- Avocado
- Extra virgin coconut oil
- Unrefined cold pressed oils like olive oil, flax seed, or sesame oil
- Wild caught fish like wild caught pacific salmon, wild sardines, or wild mackerel

Other healing foods that heal your hormones:

- Quinoa with ghee butter
- Organic eggs, sunny side up or soft-boiled for two minutes to keep the yolk soft

- Dark green veggies
- Bright colored veggies
- Spices and herbs like cinnamon, ginger, and turmeric

So, get to loving your hormones and start balancing them with some wonderful and delicious foods. And because of balanced hormones your gut inflammation will also subside.

How can I do gentle detoxifying colon cleanses?

If you want to do a natural colon and GI cleanse without harsh products, your best bet will be cleansing using nutrition. You can do that by adding great natural antiseptic (natural anti-microbial) foods like:

- Oregano oil
- Turmeric
- Onion
- Garlic
- Raw pumpkin seeds
- Cloves
- Extra virgin coconut oil
- Apple cider vinegar
- Thyme
- Green onion
- Raw carrot juice
- Pomegranate
- Horseradish

How much is enough of the natural detox foods?

You want to make sure that you eat at least four servings of the above-mentioned foods daily. Again, these are the types of foods you may want to try after the flare. It's always good to calm down the stomach first. And always speak with your health care professional, if you are ready for this.

Can your food be used as detox?

In a way, eating a certain food can become detoxifying. That can happen because the adrenals are more balanced, which will cool down the inflammation. And now inflammation is no longer stopping your body from the detoxing.

Start your detox by adding healthy, lean, dairy-free, light proteins to all three of your meals, in addition to veggies and healthful oils like extra virgin olive oil or ghee. Keeping in mind that even proteins can be plant-based, including lentils, seeds, chia seeds, hemp seeds, spirulina, and quinoa. Rotate those with animal-based proteins for your digestive plan.

Each time you eat, your plate should contain a fist—size portion of protein, veggies double that size, and at least a spoonful of oil. Some use protein shakes to replace meals. You can certainly do that but choose them wisely. Make sure the company is reputable and its ingredients come from clean sources. The protein should be dairy-free—pea based, for example. As far as the actual detox process and purging of toxins, it should be done in the gentlest way possible.

Bone Broth

Bone broth or bone stock will be your anti-inflammatory and gut supporting and healing source of nutrients. Bone stock contains two important amino acids—proline and glycine—in addition to minerals and collagen. Proline helps strengthen cell structures and therefore helps to heal and seal leaky gut syndrome and could even help with vein walls for those having hemorrhoids. Glycine helps the detoxification process and naturally helps the body synthesize the collagen that helps in healing and improves the release of growth hormone.

You can buy bone stock or make it at home: Simply place a big bunch of bones in a crock-pot and cover them with pure, cold water. Set it to low and add two tablespoons of apple cider vinegar to the cold water to help draw the nutrients from the bones. It usually takes four hours for chicken stock and about six hours for other, harder bones. You can leave it for longer, 24 hours for chicken and 48 hours for beef. Just make sure you add enough water, since it evaporates. Season to your preference. I use garlic powder, Herbamare salt alternative, and black pepper.

How can I support the liver naturally?

You can start with a natural Light Liver Detox and can do the following:

Mix one tablespoonful of extra virgin olive oil with a little bit of freshly squeezed lemon juice. Drink that in the morning for cleansing. Drink a tablespoonful of olive oil every night around 30 minutes before going to sleep, around 10–10:30 p.m. It's a gentle way to help your liver cleanse better. And later, you can also incorporate cleansing teas into your nighttime routine. Start with dandelion tea, peppermint tea, milk thistle tea, chamomile tea, etc.

What would be a sample menu of healing foods?

Breakfast:

2–3 gluten-free and pork-free-casing turkey sausage links, 2 soft boiled eggs served with arugula & baby spinach leaves. Top with fresh chopped basil, organic non-sulphurated balsamic vinegar & olive oil.

Lunch:

Mixed green salad or sautéed spinach or arugula with slices of hormone-free chicken breast slices (4–6 oz. total), sliced stir-fried portobello mushrooms, cucumber with 1 oz. of almond ricotta cheese. Dressing made with 2 tbsp. olive oil or walnut oil, and 1 tsp. apple cider vinegar. At the end, you can have a handful of organic raspberries with 3–4 walnuts.

Dinner:
4–6 oz. of wild caught flounder topped with lemon wheels and Herbamare. Bake at 225 degrees for 15–20 minutes. Add 1–2 tbsp. of olive oil when done baking. Eat with lightly steamed asparagus and red pepper topped with 2 tsp. ghee, add in ½ of a cubed avocado. You can add half of an organic baked sweet potato.

Snack:

- Celery sticks with almond butter
- Raw carrots with hummus
- Handful of blueberries with 4–6 pecans

Anti-Inflammatory Grain Free Recipe: Grain-Free, Low Sugar or No Sugar Pumpkin Muffins (makes 6)

Ingredients
- 1 cup of organic, unsweetened pumpkin purée
- 1 egg
- 1 Tbsp. of a mixture of organic cinnamon, organic ginger, organic nutmeg and organic cloves. You can simply use cinnamon with nutmeg, if you don't have the others available
- 1 cup almond or coconut flour
- 1/2 cup Xylitol (if no SIBO present) or Stevia per your taste for no sugar option (if low sugar is your choice, you can add coconut sugar per your taste)
- 1 tsp. of organic vanilla extract

- 1/4 tsp. aluminum-free baking powder
- Sea salt, a pinch

Instructions:

1. Preheat to 350 degrees Fahrenheit. You can use silicone muffin forms or a muffin pan.
2. Mix all ingredients well.
3. Fill in about two third full.
4. Bake for 30 minutes. Let it cool after.

Some herbs that are used in the kitchen can decrease inflammation, and those include cinnamon, turmeric, cloves, ginger, and rosemary. That could become an inexpensive, anti-inflammatory help.

My recent case study:

A 39-year-old female ulcerative colitis patient came in looking for functional medicine options to work with her doctor. She was compliant with medications but still had occasional flares, suspecting food sensitivities. We addressed her inflammation with an anti-inflammatory, healing diet, and added hormone-supporting foods, removed gluten, dairy, soy and corn for her. During her first week she felt better. During the second week she felt much worse, which occasionally happens when inflammation is decreased, and the system is better at eliminating toxins. Then by weeks three and four she was improving at about 70 percent from the day she came in. We also added an adrenal program for her, and by the two-months mark she had no flares and had so much more energy.

My last note here is again about the importance of a healing diet for every single patient with digestive problem who is looking to feel better. Yes, there's a lot that can be done with modern medicine for digestive disease, but having your gut loaded with the right nutrition can be that much more helpful to set the base, the grounds, for rebuilding you a brand new healthy intestine.

What you put into your body is what you will get out in form of energy, emotions, and appearance.

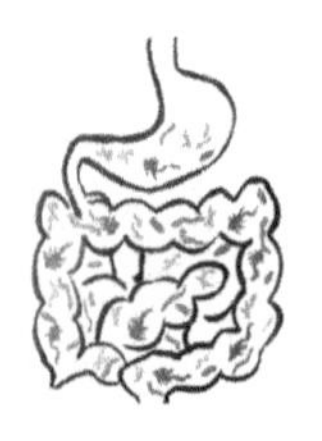

Chapter 9
FUNCTIONAL SOLUTIONS: NATURAL MEDICINES BASED ON RESEARCH

"The good thing about science is that it's true whether or not you believe in it."
– Neil deGrasse Tyson

Research Comes First

Unlike Crohn's disease, ulcerative colitis is mostly confined to the colon. Initial treatment plans for Crohn's and ulcerative colitis are very similar. Studies show that symptoms of Crohn's disease improve as the commensal bacteria becomes more diverse, although the information is still limited.

Let's talk about pharmaceutical and natural therapies. I'm a pharmacist, after all! Current treatments for Crohn's and colitis include salicylates 5-ASAs, steroids, biological agents, and surgery. Nonsteroidal anti-inflammatory agents (NSAIDS) are not effective in IBDs and it's recommended that patients with IBDs avoid using NSAIDs, since those agents impair GI healing and can potentially cause GI bleeds.

Commonly used nutraceuticals in IBDs include glutamine, iron, vitamin B6, vitamin B12, vitamin A, vitamin E, zinc, folate, aloe vera, beta glucans, n-acetyl glucosamine, psyllium, essential omega acids, NAC, GLAs, andrographis, turmeric, boswellia, colostrum, and others. Probiotics have been used in Crohn's and colitis for decades with successful results. Patients with IBDs elect to try these natural medicines because of failed attempts with traditional methods. These agents are not just popular for Crohn's and colitis, but also used for other conditions. Probiotics are living organisms of bacteria or yeast and the most common ones include Saccharomyces boulardii, Lactobacillus, and Bifidobacteria. Probiotics are introduced as "friendly" recolonizing agents and often restore the flora for patients with IBDs. These would be the agents to use if a possible root cause of IBD is related to bacterial overgrowth in the gut.

Since patients with active Crohn's or colitis have an increase number of macrophages, cytokines like interleukins, tumor necrosis factor, and lymphocytes, it becomes clear how much of an involvement there is with a broken immune system. Notice that I'm not directly calling IBD an autoimmune disease, since that has not been confirmed in the literature, but many experts suggest that it is in fact an autoimmune condition.

Most doctors would not spend more than a few minutes discussing an IBD diet with you. It's all about medication treatments. This is understandable. Doctors learn medical studies and treat according to them. Most of these serious studies are not about the diet's effect on patients. These medical studies are not about natural supplements or acupuncture treatment's effects on the patients. They are mostly about the effects of medications on the patients. That may not be because the natural and holistic treatments don't work. But that is because there's simply not enough data and studies available for the medical world to see and learn about natural or holistic treatment.

The goal in treatment for Crohn's and colitis is to keep a patient in remission (stop inflammation and prevent flare-ups). Flare-ups are the active stages of the disease with symptoms.

The main part of the treatment for IBD is medication's step-by-step protocol. These protocols are called guidelines to be followed by doctors. These guidelines are based on systemic reviews and randomized control trials. If one medication doesn't work, a doctor tries step two. If the next one fails, they will try the next line of medicine. Very often a doctor will use combinations of medications to control Crohn's/colitis symptoms. Unlike other disease guidelines, Crohn's and colitis guidelines have not been updated very often in the past twenty years. Which theoretically means that there were not that many new breakthrough drugs for IBD in the past two decades. There were many new biological medications that came on the market, but they were mostly in the similar drug category.

There are few basic categories of medications in the Crohn's disease treatment plan and I have tried most of them. I have dispensed most of them to Crohn's patients and ulcerative colitis patients and gotten enough feedback to write a book—a different book! And ulcerative colitis treatment plans look a lot like Crohn's disease treatments.

I've heard about side effects and allergies. I've heard hallucination side effect stories from a patient on Prednisone, rash side effect stories from a patient on Cipro, vomiting and diarrhea side effect stories from a patient on Flagyl, and so much more. But these medications work. They work for many patients, especially during a flare. They did work for me at my most severe state. But my idea and my mission are to make sure that you never get to the severe, life-threatening stage. And there are different ways to avoid getting there.

There's a category of medications that act as immune system suppressants, now called immunomodulators. Since in Crohn's disease our immune system is "over-reactive," these medications can reduce the immune system's reaction, but that comes with a serious side effect of immune system suppression and may be dangerous when fighting infections. It's very important to be very careful when taking these medications. The examples of these Crohn's treatments are biologicals like Humira, Remicade, Cimzia, Tysabri, etc. The older immunosuppressant is the very popular Crohn's medication called 6-MP or Mercaptopurine. There are others like Imuran, Methotrexate, Cyclosporine, etc. Methotrexate is often given for Crohn's arthritis.

One of the alternative treatments in IBD would be Low Dose Naltrexone (LDN) and alpha-lipoic acid (ALA). This combination of a drug and a nutritional supplement is looking promising and would require more analysis-based evaluations for a possible future IBD treatment. It's currently tried for cancer, IBD, Lupus and more.

IBD surgery is a last resort and has a potential for many other problems. During surgery the affected part of the intestine would be removed, leaving as much of the healthy intestine as possible. The surgery does not guarantee a positive outcome.

Treatment for IBD:

Anti-inflammatory agents

Traditional treatment: 5-ASA or 5-Aminosalicylic acid formulations or Amino salicylates. These are anti-inflammatory medications with a relatively safe side effect profile. Amino salicylate can also be used as ulcerative colitis medication, used for mild to moderate cases. 5-ASAs work as antioxidants that neutralize reactive oxygen molecules produced by neutrophils. Amino salicylates act as anti-inflammatory and prevent the production of other inflammatory mediators including leukotrienes and prostaglandins. 5-ASAs are also given to prevent flares.

- Mesalamine (Asacol, Lialda, Pentasa, Rowasa)
- Balsalazide (Colazal)
- Olsalazine (Dipentum)Sulfasalazine (Azulfidine) (increase folate intake, since the drug can inhibit the absorption of folate in the intestine)

When patients don't respond to these agents, antibiotics are often started.

Antibiotics

Traditional treatment with agents like Ciprofloxacin (Cipro) and Metronidazole (Flagyl). They are given for a short period of time. They have many side effects and they destroy the normal gut flora. Consider taking probiotics right after your antibiotics or sometimes even during the antibiotic Crohn's disease treatment. If you decide to take it during the antibiotic therapy, consider spacing antibiotics and probiotics about 2–3 hours apart to avoid interactions.

In moderate to severe cases, corticosteroids may be tried. They are also offered to those with mild cases of IBD that do not respond to 5-ASAs. The classic one is Prednisone. It's very potent. It has many side effects and is usually given for a short time. There's also Budesonide, which has fewer side effects because its delivery system is more local. Lots of patients don't like to use steroids because of their side effect profile, which includes behavioral changes, sleeplessness, moon face, and many more. Many would like to opt out for more natural options without harsh side effects.

Natural Medicines:

- Bromelain, used for improving digestion
- Andrographis (Andrographis paniculate), used for improving the immune system
- Essential fatty acids like alpha-linolenic acid, conjugated linoleic acid and evening primrose oil, used for decreasing inflammation
- Fish oil, including Docosahexaenoic acid (DHA) and Eicosapentaenoic (EPA), used for decreasing inflammation
- Gamma linolenic acid, used for hormone-balancing and decreasing inflammation
- Colostrum, used for balancing the immune system
- Bovine IgG (dairy-free immunoglobulin), used for balancing the immune system
- Rutin, used for its antioxidant properties
- Green tea (Camellia sinensis), used for antioxidant effect
- Wheatgrass (Elytrigia repens), used for detoxification
- Indian frankincense (Boswellia serrata), used for inflammation
- Turmeric (Curcuma longa), used for decreasing inflammation
- Phosphatidylcholine, used for anti-inflammatory effect

Immunomodulators

Immunomodulators are used in IBD patients that don't respond to steroids. They cool down the inflammation and immune system response. Azathioprine or mercaptopurine are effective in remission and a flare of Crohn's disease. These medications are also used in colitis. Methotrexate is sometimes used for Crohn's disease, probably less now than before. Cyclosporine is used for severe colitis. Cyclosporine can be a rescue for those not responding to steroids who want to avoid surgery. In Crohn's disease this medication doesn't seem to be effective.

Immunomodulators are often used for IBD patients who don't respond to or can't tolerate other treatments. Golimumab is used to achieve and maintain remission in patients with moderate-to-severe active colitis. Adalimumab and certolizumab are effective in decreasing symptoms and keeping moderate to severe Crohn's patients in remission. Infliximab is used in patients with both types of IBD.

Natalizumab and vedolizumab are given to those that can't tolerate other therapies and for moderate to severe Crohn's patients to maintain remission. Vedolizumab is used in patients with active IBD. Ustekinumab are also used to treat IBD and it helps decrease symptoms and maintain remission in patients with moderate to severe active Crohn's.

Traditional Medications:

- 6-Mercaptopurine (Purinethol, Purixan)
- Infliximab (Remicade)
- Methotrexate (Rheumatrex)
- Natalizumab (Tysabri)
- Ustekinumab (Stelara)
- Vedolizumab (Entyvio)
- Adalimumab (Humira)
- Azathioprine (Azasan, Imuran)
- Certolizumab (Cimzia)
- Cyclosporine (Gengraf, Neoral, Sandimmune)
- Golimumab (Simponi)

Natural Medicines

Probiotics:

- Lactobacillus
- Bifidobacteria
- Saccharomyces boulardii

Nutrients:

- Iron
- Vitamin A
- Vitamin B6
- Vitamin B12
- Glutamine
- Vitamin E
- Zinc

Other natural medicines used for IBD:

- Peppermint (*Mentha x piperita*)
- N-acetyl glucosamine
- Wheat bran (*Triticum aestivum*)
- Aloe gel (*Aloe vera*)
- Barley (*Hordeum vulgare*)
- Beta glucans
- Blond psyllium (*Plantago ovata*)

Treating IBD is a long process and now as many as half of IBD patients are looking for natural medicines because their symptoms are not relieved. And many of those patients use them on top of their traditional therapies, often without mentioning it to their doctors. That can create all sort of problems, including drug—herb interaction, food—herb interaction, enhanced activity of the drug, decreased activity of the drug, and many more. Following up with a professional that can do all those checks for you is extremely important.

Drugs used for diarrhea in IBD are loperamide and diphenoxylate. Sometimes abdominal pain and cramping are treated with older medications such as belladonna, dicyclomine, and propantheline. It's important not to use those medications for severe cases of colitis because in those cases it's crucial to seek emergency help.

Omega Fish oil is often tried for colitis and Crohn's. Fish oil contains the omega-3 fatty acids eicosapentaenoic acid (EPA) and docosahexaenoic acid (DHA). Fish oil has anti-inflammatory and immunomodulatory effects and it suppresses mediators of immune function.

Fish oil has been studied for Crohn's in small clinical trials and the results are inconsistent. Two meta-analyses assessed results from six clinical trials that include over one thousand patients with Crohn's. Results show that treatment with omega fish oil may decrease the relapse rate of Crohn's disease by 13% compared to a placebo. Larger clinical trials show that taking omega fish oils will not decrease symptoms but may decrease the need for steroids.

Other oils were studied for IBD. The combination of evening primrose oil and borage oil taken for five months may improve stool consistency in patients with colitis, but didn't seem to influence stool frequency, rectal bleeding, or disease relapse. It's important to use a quality omega oil, and the ratio omega 6 to omega 3 should be 3:1 at most, since Omega 6 oils in excess are associated with potential risks.

Blond psyllium was studied for colitis and Crohn's. Fermentation of psyllium in the GI tract produces butyrate that has an anti-inflammatory effect. There was preliminary clinical evidence that taking blond psyllium 10 grams twice daily can be as effective as mesalamine 500 mg three times daily for preventing relapse of ulcerative colitis. Blond psyllium also appears to help relieve many of the GI symptoms of ulcerative colitis, including abdominal pain, bloating, and diarrhea. But it didn't work in younger patients. It also has been studied in Crohn's, in a study where it was found that taking blond psyllium 9.9 grams daily along with a lacto and bifido probiotic seems to decrease the index disease activity in people with Crohn's disease. But we are not yet sure if it's the probiotic, the psyllium or both.

Probiotics for IBDs:

Crohn's and colitis practice guidelines depend on older trials, while new information is very well worth investigating. Ulcerative colitis guidelines recognize the benefit of probiotic VSL#3 for pouchitis, while Crohn's disease guidelines are still cautious about recommending them.

There's more research done on probiotic use in ulcerative colitis than for Crohn's disease. But, even the limited data in Crohn's studies shows a lot of promise. Some data suggests that S. Boulardii can decrease the frequency of diarrhea in Crohn's patients. Some preliminary clinical studies for Crohn's disease suggests that S. Boulardii (Saccharomyces Boulardii), taken as 1 gram once daily combined with mesalamine, taken as1 gram twice daily, after 6 months of treatment, will have a decreased rate of relapse when comparing to only the mesalamine patient group. However, other data suggests that using Lactobacillus johnsonii strand was not effective in preventing flare ups after surgery in Crohn's disease.

Some clinical investigation shows that VSL#3 can prevent pathogenic growth and improve condition of ulcerative colitis patients, who can't take mesalamines, by preventing relapse. There's also some research showing that combining VSL#3 with traditional therapy including balsalazide improves remission when it's compared to therapy with mesalamine alone or balsalazide alone in patients that have mild to moderate ulcerative colitis.

Pediatric patients with active moderate to severe ulcerative colitis who are taking VSL#3 with salicylates can increase their remission rate up to 92.8% and decrease their flare ups by 68%. Other research shows that adding VSL#3 in patients with active mild to moderate ulcerative colitis, who don't respond to traditional therapy, can initiate remission in up to 53% of patients. VSL#3 can also help in treating chronic pouchitis, which can be a complication of surgery. When VSL#3 was used continuously for one year it helped maintain remission in 85% of patients.

Preliminary evidence shows that S. Boulardii can help UC as well. Adding S. Boulardii, at a dose of 250mg three times daily, can decrease symptoms in mild and moderate UC cases in those patients who still have exacerbations being on mesalamine alone.

As a recommendation, it seems that probiotics can be an advantageous addition to current treatment plans. It's more especially suggested to use S. Boulardii for Crohn's disease patients. But, VSL#3 can possibly be very effective if used for a longer period, like one year. Symbiotic agents (probiotic plus prebiotic) also have good data that starts indicating them for Crohn's patients with possible bacterial overgrowth or permeability problems. And lastly, testing microbiology for commensal bacteria in Crohn's patients is a good start for evaluating the gut flora of an IBD patient. When there is a need for an anti-inflammatory probiotic, F. prausnitzii would be beneficial.

Patients on conventional immunosuppressants, such as methotrexate and cyclosporine, should probably avoid use of probiotics, especially Lactobacillus types, to avoid the rare possibility of pathogenic colonization. With an educated practitioner you will be able to decide when you will be ready to start.

Many multi-probiotic blends have common ingredient blends. Following are those good probiotic ingredients you often see on the labels:

- **Bifidobacterium Lactis**: Take this to improve symptoms of diarrhea, to repopulate after depletion, or after antibiotic use, etc.
- **Bifidobacterium Bifidum:** Take this to protect your microbiome from serious cases of diarrhea, protecting it from pathogenic overgrowth.
- **Bifidobacterium Longum**: Take this to restore flora. Our lining is covered with it when we are born, but we lose it over the years, especially if our diet isn't feeding this good bacterium.

- **Bacillus Subtilis**: Take this for regularity, nausea, upset stomach, gas, bloating, etc.
- **Lactobacillus Rhamnosus**: Take this to protect lining from overgrowth of pathogens.
- **Lactobacillus Acidophilus**: Take this to help with diarrhea and improve digestion.
- **Lactobacillus Casei**: Take this for a quick relief of diarrhea, etc.
- **Lactobacillus Plantarum**: Take this when flatulence is your main symptom.
- **Lactobacillus Gasseri**: Take this to improve metabolic syndrome issues.
- **Lactobacillus Paracasei**: Take this when your body is having a hard time breaking down certain sugars in packaged, processed foods.
- **Streptococcus Thermophilus**: Take this when you have trouble with dairy foods, since it helps with enzymatic activity. Note, though, that many IBD patients have trouble with this ingredient since it causes them GI irritability.

Nutraceuticals

Colostrum

Colostrum provides a perfect combination of immune and growth factors including immunoglobulins, lactoferrin and insulin-like growth factor 1 (IGF-1) or colostrum transfer factor. And it also provides the perfect blend of amino acids and other natural immune boosting properties.

Bovine derived IgG (immunoglobulins)

The discovery that the gut barrier plays a key role in immune health fueled the search to strengthen it. In that search, researchers found that the binding capabilities of immunoglobulins have a positive effect on gut barrier function. Immunoglobulins bind microbes and toxins in the GI tract and eliminate them prior to immune system activation. As these unwanted triggers are removed, it resets healthy immune tolerance and builds a stronger barrier to the external environment.

Turmeric

Turmeric is a yellow spice from the ginger family. Curcumin is the active ingredient of turmeric. Research shows that curcumin has anti-inflammatory activity, possibly by inhibiting COX-2, prostaglandins, leukotrienes, and other cytokines. A small study shows that taking curcumin 1.08 grams daily for one month followed by 1.44 grams daily for another month decreases diarrhea and stomach pain compared to baseline in patients with Crohn's. There's some research using curcumin in patients with ulcerative colitis. A clinical study shows that taking curcumin 1.1 grams daily for one month followed by 1.65 grams daily for another month decreases symptoms of ulcerative colitis in patients taking mesalamines and corticosteroids compared to baseline.

Another natural medicine used by patients with IBD is andrographis, which has immunostimulant properties. Andrographis inhibits tumor necrosis factor (TNF)-alpha, interleukin (IL)-1beta, and nuclear factor (NF)-κB, proving that it has anti-inflammatory properties. In a small trial, andrographis was taken as an extract 1,200 to 1,800 mg daily for eight weeks and decreased symptoms of mild to moderate colitis compared to a placebo. More research is needed but the agent looks promising.

Many nutrients are used to treat IBD. L-glutamine is an amino acid that is sometimes used in Crohn's. Depletion of glutamine can result in damage to the intestinal lining. There's some data showing evidence that glutamine affects GI cell proliferation and differentiation, and more studies are needed.

Patients with Crohn's and colitis often try natural anti-inflammatories. Bromelain is considered an enzymatic natural anti-inflammatory agent. Bromelain is a proteolytic enzyme found in pineapple.

Rutin is a flavonoid that seems to work similarly to an antioxidant effect of mesalamines. There are animal studies of the anti-inflammatory effect of rutin in colitis.

Indian frankincense, also known as boswellia, contains the anti-inflammatory agents boswellic acid and alpha-boswellic acid. Some data indicates that Indian frankincense gum resin 350 mg three times daily might induce remission of ulcerative colitis.

Phosphatidylcholine is a phospholipid that can be derived from soy, sunflower, and mustard. It can also come from eggs. Phosphatidylcholine is thought to have anti-inflammatory effects and colon protective effects. Clinical research suggests that taking slow-release, phosphatidylcholine-rich phospholipids 6 grams daily for 3 months improves the rate of remission and improves the symptoms compared to placebo in patients with colitis.

Green tea contains catechins that might have anti-inflammatory activity and possibly benefit patients with IBD. Preliminary clinical research suggests that taking a specific green tea product can help achieve remission in patients with colitis.

Aloe Vera has an antioxidant effect, decreasing levels of colorectal prostaglandin E2 and interleukin-8, and because of the mechanism of action it has garnered attention for a possibility in treating IBD. There have been some results so far but not enough information is available yet. Aloe latex is another aloe plant product and can be irritating to the gut lining. Although it's found in many alternative preparations I wouldn't recommend it for many patients for that reason.

Glutathione. What is Glutathione? Glutathione is a very important antioxidant. It is abbreviated as GSH. Glutathione is a type of a small protein that is essential to your health. Living organisms could not survive without GSH. Some amino acids are needed to make GSH. Those are GSH's precursors called glutamic acid, cysteine, and glycine. One common natural supplement that many Crohn's disease patients take is called N-Acetyl-Cysteine (NAC), which is derived from the amino acid L-Cysteine.

Taking this supplement can increase the levels of GSH. But there are other great products available that improve GSH levels. It is almost impossible to boost the levels of GSH by eating certain foods. So, to get it you would need to obtain supplements from a trusted source. There is research literature available on PubMed if you would like to learn more.

It's very important to remember that all-natural medicines are still medicines and it is best to have a practitioner that knows your entire list, including the traditional and alternative/complementary medications.

Basic and General Nutraceutical Protocol for IBD Support:

Do not try new supplements without discussing them with your physician or healthcare practitioner first.

- Immune Support (ex, Colostrum by DFH) or Bovine IgG (ex, SBI Protect by OrthoMolecularProducts) 1-2 capsules twice daily
- Probiotics (ex, Probiospheres (DFH) or MultiProbiotics (Garden of Life Original Medicine Line)) 1 capsule once to twice daily and S. Boulardii 1 capsule once daily
- Multipacks with active B complex and Omega/vitD/vitK 1 packet twice daily
- L-Glutamine 1 Tbsp. once daily

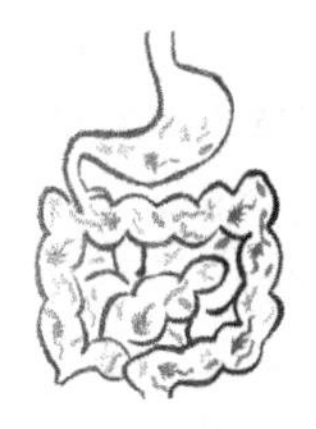

Chapter 10
FUNCTIONAL SOLUTIONS: DETOXIFICATION

"My own prescription for health is less paperwork and more running barefoot through the grass"
– Leslie Grimutter

Why Would You Be Toxic?

If you are like most people, you don't think about how pollution, toxicity at home, and a toxic mind is affecting you every day. As health care professionals we are also not trained to determine the extent of the damage, nor are we trained to teach our patients to protect themselves from harsh environmental effects.

Many of the products labeled "natural," "eco-friendly," and "green" still contain toxins. So it's important to get educated.

Let's talk air pollution. We spend so much time at home, and indoor air quality is just terrible. Depending on each home we can find mixtures of volatile organic compounds (VOCs) emitted as vapor into the home air from things like carpet, cleaning products, plastics, paints, electronic equipment, and cosmetics. Gas heaters can cause elevated levels of carbon dioxide. VOCs are associated with cancers and other harmful health effects.

While air filters are surely an option, you can do a great thing for your home air using house plants. This is an inexpensive natural way to detox your home.

- Highly recommended plants to improve air quality include:
- Boston Fern
- Spider Plant
- Peace Lily
- Common Ivy
- Bamboo Plant
- Lady Palm
- English Ivy
- Rubber Plants
- African Violets
- Palm Tree
- Gerbera Daisy

Plastics and Phthalates

Phthalates were supposed to make the plastics better and softer. They're now commonly used in vinyl flooring, blinds, shower curtains, plastic wraps, food containers, kids' lunch boxes, beauty products, nail polish, car parts, kids' toys, kids' electronic devices, household cleaners, and many more plastic products.

They are also used in sprays, gels, and air fresheners. Even natural labels may contain them. Let's get educated and remove them from the home, because the heavier the toxic and chemical load is in your home, the more your body gets polluted. It's possible to get chronic problems with toxin burden.

What makes phthalates even more problematic for Crohn's and colitis patients is the fact that they are present in the enteric coatings of certain drugs and some nutritional supplements. They can also be found in gelling agents, film formers, lubricants, suspensions, and emulsifiers. They can be found in catheters and even blood transfusion devices. And IBD patients spend time in the hospital more than an average person. A study from Harvard School of Public Health from 2004 found that enteric coating used on drugs and some supplements have polymers that contain plasticizers, including phthalates. The study included information on a man who started Asacol (enteric coated medication, commonly used in Crohn's and colitis). His urine was collected three months after initiating the medication and the results showed that the concentration of phthalates was higher than most men surveyed in the 1999 to 2000 National Health and Nutrition Examination Survey. Now would be a good time to start cleaning up unnecessary ingredients from drugs and nutraceuticals.

Germs All over Your Home

Do you wear your outside shoes inside your home? If you do, you may be bringing an entire chemical and microbiology lab into your home, including strep and staph bacteria, allergens, viruses, mold, even lead and much more. Leave your shoes at the door.

Dust and More Air Pollution

If you are not allergic to dust, you may not notice the harmful effects of accumulated dust. By removing your shoes, you can reduce the amount of dust in your home by half.

Candles used at home are also associated with air pollution, especially the cheaper kind. Paraffin costs much less than beeswax. So, most candles are made from paraffin. Paraffin is a toxic waste product made from petroleum. Stay away from those and only consider using the candles labeled "made from beeswax."

You know you should probably switch to nontoxic cleaners, but without the understanding of why, it's hard to get the motivation to do it. After all, the cleaners you buy usually say they're "green" or "natural," so they can't be all bad, right? They can't really give you diseases, right? The bad news is, they can be all bad for *you*, even if they are not "bad" for the environment.

Problems with Cleaning Products

Many, if not most, cleaning products are not tested for safety. That will need to come to an end soon. Chlorine or other chemical containing cleaning products used in most American homes can potentially have detrimental health effects if used for a long period of time. Read the labels and know what's in your cleaning products. There are companies that make safer and more eco friendly cleaning products.

Fluoride is another chemical that is found in so many products, including dental products, cleaners, and public water. Fluoride is associated with bone cancer, joint pain, thyroid damage, mental and physiological changes, and more. Consider switching your toothpaste to one that's fluoride-free.

BPA, or bisphenol A, is used in plastics and is a chemical associated with hormone disruptions, baby development issues, and more. Products labeled BPA—free are often substituted with BPS, an equally toxic chemical. So, opt-in for glass or quality stainless steel containers for your kids and yourself.

Preservatives such as parabens and PEG have issues associated with hormone disruptions, onset of early puberty, cancers, fertility issues, and many more. Investigate paraben-free products and read labels to make sure no other substitution chemical was snuck in. You don't need to be a pharmacist to recognize paraben ingredients such methyparaben, ethylparaben, butylparaben, benzylparaben, isobutylparaben, and isopropylparaben. Avoid those like the plague.

Aluminum in many deodorants is associated with the risk of breast cancer, allergies, hormonal imbalances, birth defects, and more. There are natural deodorants on the market that contain only natural ingredients and do not cause clogged lymph nodes and health problems.

Homemade Deodorant Ingredients:

- 1 tbsp. cocoa butter
- 1 tbsp. coconut oil
- 2 1/2 tbsp. arrowroot powder
- 1 tbsp. baking soda
- 1/4 tsp. gluten-free vitamin E oil
- 15 drops essential oil of your choice

Melt cocoa butter and coconut oil over low heat. Remove the pot from heat, then add arrowroot powder and baking soda. Mix it up until all powders are dissolved and combined. Add vitamin E oil and essential oils. Allow mixture to cool in pan. Place in refrigerator to cool and harden. After this, the product may be stored on counter. Use just a little bit and spread.

The following are ingredients you should avoid at all costs:

- mineral oil
- SLS (sodium lauryl sulfate)
- paraffin
- parabens, including parahydroxybenzoate, butylparaben, methylparaben, propylparaben, and ethylparaben

- unspecified "fragrance" or "flavor"
- oxybenzone
- butylated hydroxytoluene (BHT)
- diazolidinyl urea
- octinoxate/ethylhexyl methoxycinnamate (this is a sunscreen ingredient)
- propylene glycol

The market is growing for cleaner sun protection options. And the safest ingredient for natural sunscreen is Zinc Oxide. I like using products by the company named Badger. I use it on my children because the ingredients are so clean. EWG.org is the environmental working group that has the newest updates on companies that make clean sunscreen. They also have the dirty dozen and the clean fifteen information every year. That includes produce with the twelve most hormone-altering disrupters and the fifteen cleanest vegetables and fruits each year. Following this great website is a good time saver when looking for cleaner products and cleaner produce.

Detoxing your mind may seem easier said than done. It's easy to say "just go home and meditate and you'll feel better," but what about those who can't meditate and just can't shut off their mind? What about those who don't believe in all this?

I know that it's hard to bring your attention to breath when your stomach hurts like crazy. And I know that when you have a fever and your body shakes madly it's not realistic to sit down to do EFT. So, I've trained myself to do those things at those moments when I was feeling better. And in the beginning, it was hard. Because the moment you feel better you want to have fun or watch TV or simply enjoy yourself. But once you get to realize that detoxing your mind is not hard work and not a chore, but a fun activity that will get you healthier then you will want to do more and more of it.

A few things you want to do to detox your mind:

First, stop absorbing the news. If you pay close attention, more negative news is available on TV and in social media. Create an environment where you are not fed negativity. Choose to watch a Netflix movie of your choice without interruptions or cancer treatment commercials.

Second, flood your mind with positivity. It's not easy when your symptoms are severe. But if you can find one good thing about today, you can start finding more and more each day. Start by thinking how good you have it compared to someone living with no heat, no light, and no future. Your life is amazing!

Third, give up your coffee. This one isn't easy to do. But so worth it. This should be a slow tapering process, but once you are completely caffeine—free, your adrenals will thank you and your mind won't depend on chemicals to keep it happy.

Fourth, do not overthink and do not question your treatment over and over. Do not try to be your own doctor. Yes, be your own patient advocate, but it's not possible to be your own doctor. It just doesn't work. Even the best doctors go to another healthcare professional.

Fifth, jump out your bed in the morning with an intention for a good day. Set your intentions right away for a symptom-free day, for finding a better doctor that suits you, to find a better food place near you that has paleo and gluten-free options, etc. You control what you think and if you think positively, your gut and your body will catch on.

Get up and get to work on a goal, a project, or a specific task.

A negative result of overthinking is that it slows you down, inhibiting your growth, limiting your ability to have love, good relationships, fun in the moment, and pursuit of success in business or career.

One tip that I've learned that did more than detox my mind from overthinking is to turn my often-worrisome thoughts about the future into effort and work. Acting, moving, doing something, and working on what you love does wonders for your soul.

Each time I would start to worry about the future, I would make a conscious decision to physically get up from where I was sitting and start walking to actually do something like working on my book or other materials. Sometimes I would go outside to simply take a quick walk. Planting veggies in the backyard is so de-stressing and I know my clients swear by this planting therapy. If I was working, I would start jotting down some writing ideas on how to improve my work or simply work on something that I love. Whatever the task you choose, make sure it is a difficult task because that's when you start to get that energy flow or momentum. That's the place where you get most of your happy moments. Detoxing the mind is done to simply feel good. And feeling good is our birthright. Accept what is. Do not overthink. Continue and love the chaos.

Constipation as a problem in IBDs related to toxins.

In cases of chronic constipation with IBD patients, we are often concerned with inflammation that makes the intestines swell up, so the passage becomes more narrow. This can create blockages. When constipation is persistent in the case of IBD, we are not just concerned with pain, bloating, gasses, and mostly uncomfortable symptoms, but we are concerned with developing more serious problems like diverticulitis, gut microbiome changes, rectal prolapse, and fissures. Preventing constipation should become an unquestionable duty. And occasional colon cleansing should be considered.

Colon Cleanse Questions:

"I have Crohn's disease and I want to cleanse my colon and liver together and am considering a total colon cleanse, should I go with OTC products or should I see a professional?"

And as always, I advise that you see a health care professional. It can be a doctor, naturopath or other holistic practitioner. But it must be someone with lots of credibility.

We realize that for a healthy body we need a healthy and "clean" colon.

We need to love our "gut" to get its love back. The intestinal tract is very complex. Our intestinal tract (gut) has many nerve endings, which let you know that something is wrong with pain signals to the brain. And boy, the kind of stomach pain that can be sometimes....

The intestinal tract is responsible for many things, including the extremely important part of removing the waste out of our digestive system.

What happens if the digestive system encounters a problem? The digestive system may "back up," "overflow" and cause nausea, vomiting, constipation and even rebound diarrhea. That's not the worst part yet. It gets worse when all those toxins get back (reabsorbed) into the bloodstream, poisoning your entire system.

The cycle of health starts from the healthy liver. When the liver is healthy, so is the colon. Normally, the liver will try to clean itself of these toxins by means of sweat, urine, and stool.

But, when it gets too toxic, the liver will throw toxins into other organs—like skin for example. Skin is the largest organ on our body. So, many patients will experience skin problems like eczema, acne, rosacea, and others because of digestive problems. And most doctors won't tell you that the skin issues are coming from your digestive problems.

Some people may also have newly developed allergies because the liver is so overwhelmed that it can't remove any more "foreign particles."

I can't say enough that the liver is an extremely important part of the digestive system. A liver cleanse is sometimes paired with a colon cleanse for better detoxification results.

Colon Cleanse Questions:

What do we use for a super colon cleansing?

I'd like to first let you know all the things that you should probably not use for colon detox. Those would be the over the counter laxatives like Senna, Fleet Phospho-Soda, Dulcolax (Bisacodyl), and many more.

These are fine for occasional constipation but even then, they should be used with caution because of the side effects and all that cramping. They are too harsh and can be abrasive to the colon.

When using these laxatives for a prolonged time they can cause a condition called Melanosis coli that is an indication of bowel dependency or "lazy colon syndrome." The patient will develop a so-called dependency and will need to always continue the laxative.

Constipation is a big problem, especially in the summer. You may be more dehydrated from the heat causing the colon to lose the water.

Symptoms of constipation will present in inability to move bowels, gas, stomach pain, and sometimes even nausea and vomiting. It's important to recognize symptoms of constipation early because chronic constipation can lead to serious secondary digestive conditions.

There are many kinds of foods that cause constipation in adults and children. Foods that cause constipation can include potatoes, chocolate, white bread, pasta, and many more. Overeating any food and not chewing food enough can also make you more constipated. Make sure to chew well.

Chronic constipation is an issue for so many people. One of the more serious concerns is that many people don't even know they have chronic constipation, thinking going to the bathroom twice a week is okay. You need to go at least once to two times a day!

The original Master Cleanse was thought to be developed in the 1940s and it takes 10–16 days for the cleanse to really take effect.

Ingredients (single serving):

- 2 tbsp.organic lemon juice (1/2 lemon)
- 2 tbsp.organic maple syrup (grade B; not the commercial maple flavored syrup served on pancakes)—you can buy it in any health food store
- 1/10 tsp. cayenne pepper powder
- 10 ounces filtered water

Preparation: Mix all the ingredients together. Drink the liquid 5–8 times a day for at least 10 days.

Other Options for Safe Colon Cleanses:

- You can occasionally do juice cleansing days, where you only drink juices. This in return would let the digestive system relax and as a result you can get improved peristalsis. That's not an option for those with blood sugar instability.
- You can do some colon cleanses with essential oils, using peppermint, lemon and honey.
- For a very gentle cleanse, try oil pulling. Two ways: (1) fill your mouth with olive oil and hold it there for a couple of minutes before swirling it around the mouth and spitting it out. The process shouldn't exceed more than three or four minutes; it's repeated at least two or three times weekly; or (2) for those that feel nauseous, try holding coconut or extra virgin olive oil still in the mouth for three to five minutes. Then spit out the liquid.
- Some love cleansing with flax mill. To do so, in place of your morning meal, eat this mixture for three weeks:
    - Week One: 1 tablespoon of freshly milled flax seeds and 100 ml of cultured coconut milk or kefir

- Week Two: 2 tablespoons of freshly milled flax seeds and 100 ml of cultured coconut milk or kefir
- Week Three: 3 tablespoons of freshly milled flax seeds and 150 ml of cultured coconut milk or kefir
- Make a new portion of milled flax seeds every morning. This will prevent it from going bad and it will keep more nutrients when freshly milled.
- Remember to drink at least two liters of water a day.

Options for Diarrhea

While over the counter options are available and effective for diarrhea, you don't want to rely on them all the time. Those include: Imodium (loperamide), Kaopectate, and PeptoBismol. Addressing root causes, anxiety, inflammation, and food sensitivities are important steps for stopping chronic diarrhea. And there are natural options available, like psyllium, activated charcoal, bentonite magma, and homeopathic preps for diarrhea like the one from the company HEEL.

Liver Flush

I am the biggest fan of liver flushing and do them myself. But I must warn you, you may not like me the night you are doing one. Or you can be the one that lets me know that it was a piece of cake! This is for your information only and if you decide to try it, always discuss with your health care practitioner first.

Supplies:

1. Two ounces of freshly squeezed lemon juice. (1–2 lemons)
2. Ultra Phos liquid. It's really beneficial to use it to soften the bile stones.
3. Olive oil. Regular extra virgin oil will do.
4. Coca Cola Classic. Bottle, *not* can. (Yes, it can be a plastic bottle.)

5. Apple Cider or Unfiltered Apple Juice. It's better if it's organic apple cider, but just regular old apple cider you can get at the grocery store is fine. Organic unfiltered, unprocessed apple juice works too.

Do not eat a lot of protein for three days—mostly fruits and vegetables, please. You can continue the diet freely, though. No need to fast.

For three days, drink one quart of apple cider per day. Add 90 drops of Ultra Phos liquid to each quart before you start drinking the juice. You can drink the apple cider throughout the day. With meals, between meals, it doesn't matter. On the third day of drinking the apple cider, at least three hours after your evening meal, you do the liver flush.

Mix together the following:

- 2 ounces of freshly squeezed lemon juice, usually 1 full lemon
- 4 ounces of unrefined extra virgin olive oil or unrefined sesame oil.
- 4 ounces of Coke from the glass bottle or regular bottle, not from a can. Don't use other types of Coke, specifically the original classic. (Shake the Coke a few times to get all the fizz out). I know Coke isn't the best thing for you, but doing this flush can be so detoxing. So, it's better to use Coke once just to be able to get a cup of oil down and keep it down. You may become nauseous if you don't.

Stir this mixture together. Do not shake. Stir vigorously, then drink.

After drinking, lay down on your right side right away, knees slightly bent, head properly supported, at least for 30 minutes. Then spend 15 minutes on your left side and 15 minutes on your back. Start moving around. Do not have a lot of activities that night. Try to rest. You must go to sleep at 10 p.m.

Results: The oil usually passes within a good few hours. Be prepared to get up at night to go to the bathroom. If you experience any nausea, treat it with ginger or peppermint tea. The nausea leaves once the oil has passed. Within 12 to 24 hours the debris that was congesting in the liver will pass. Green, pea size stones, dead parasites, and lymphatic debris. Drink plenty of distilled water over the next few days.

The effects of the liver flush can be so rewarding. You are literally cleaning your body's blood filter. When you want to heal completely, you want to clean the "filters."

It's very beneficial to do a liver flush after an anti-parasitic program that can be generally recommended—or better yet, recommended to you specifically after a good PCR based stool test. You can do it again as maintenance twice a year. You'll be surprised at how good you will feel.

Lymphatic Detoxification

Lymphatic detoxification is not getting enough attention and it can be particularly useful for chronic digestive sufferers. Over the past 80 years more than 70,000 industrial chemicals have been created and are now part of our environment. These toxins are found in our food, air and water. Add other toxins to the mix—alcohol, medications, excess coffee, and smoking—and now you can understand why we are unwell, sluggish, sleepless, depressed, have low energy, and are overweight.

The lymphatic system aids the immune system in removing and destroying waste, debris, dead blood cells, pathogens, toxins, and cancer cells. It also helps to absorb fats and fat-soluble vitamins from the digestive system and deliver these nutrients to the cells of the body where they are used. The lymphatic system also removes excess fluid and waste products from the interstitial spaces between the cells.

If the lymphatic system is overwhelmed and sluggish, how could it perform the job properly? The lymphatic system is a detoxification system and is responsible for clearing toxins that cause diseases. Some clues that you may have a compromised lymph system are pain in the underarm area, groin area, behind the ears, or in the neck area. A common symptom that most people have experienced is swollen glands during a viral or bacterial infection.

What can be done to improve lymphatic drainage?

1. Drink plenty of fluids, water (two liters) to prevent thickening of the lymph fluid
2. Go regularly to saunas to sweat it out
3. Do contrast showers (hot alternating with cold) to promote the movement of the lymph
4. Dry brushing (always have the flow towards your heart)
5. See a professional lymphatic detox specialist
6. Move, exercise, or rebound to move lymph to cleanse
7. Complex homeopathy that focuses on drainage

Detoxing your Relationships

No master cleanse can improve your toxic relationships. We investigate model behavior on TV and social media. We investigate our friends' and our neighbors' relationships as something to copy. We develop the need for approval from others and from society. And that's how it becomes okay to stay in a toxic relationship.

Although it's hard and scary for some people to be alone without a partner, many realize that it's better to be alone than spend your time with someone who makes you sick, literally.

Toxic relationships bring fears, anxiety, depression, despair, jealousy, and all the negative emotions that IBD patients cannot stomach—yes, literally. Getting the relationship fixed is one great solution, except most really can't do it alone and need help. They should seek help because it will also be healing physically.

It's very important to surround yourself with people that are positive, encouraging, honest, and grateful. And learning the steps of getting to a healthier relationship is a big key to success here.

First, remind yourself how much you are worth to yourself—not how much you are worth to your partner or your friend! It's so important to remember that your health depends on your love for yourself. If you don't love yourself, you will eat unhealthily, and your health will suffer. If you don't love yourself, you will not do what's good for your body, and that's not good for your health.

Get into the habit of praising yourself for little and big things. You woke up and made your bed. Yes, success. I'm starting with success today. You walked for 15 minutes today. Yes, success. I got oxygen into my lungs and moved my lymph. What a great thing I did today for myself. Do it with fun, love for yourself, and excitement and notice how you can turn into the most positive person, over time with practice.

Second, sometimes negative relationships need to go, or your health will go. Stop and think about if your relationships with friends, relatives and partners are causing you a lot of pain. If it's a relationship that must come to an end, then it may be the healthiest thing you can do for your body. Ideally, that should be done with the help of a therapist.

Choosing relationships that are positive, encouraging, and energizing will be life-changing. Set high standards for yourself, talk through and release negative emotions and commit to spending the most amount of your time with those who affect you in a positive way.

What would be a good detox for an entire system including kidney cleanse, liver cleanse, blood cleanse, and colon cleanse?

If your approach to kidney cleanse is with food, then you must start with cranberries, blueberries, and black cherries for at least two weeks. Get into the habit of regularly adding unsweetened cranberry juice into your water, drink celery juice, and consider Organic Tulsi Liver and Kidney Support Tea, which has a powerful herbal combination to cleanse.

Using beets for kidney and blood has been the staple in European recipes. Pickled or fermented beets can be added to your diet. Or, use beet juice which is high in nitric oxide and is very helpful in cleansing the blood.

I can't give enough praise to the benefits of drinking warm water with freshly squeezed lemon juice in the morning. It helps with detoxification and alkalinity. Lemon juice is even recommended for prevention of kidney stones.

Your day of blood and kidney cleanse can look like this:

Breakfast: Smoothie with half a cup of frozen cherries, blueberries, and cranberries with added dairy-free protein mix and flax milk. You can add your favorite greens in there too.

Lunch: Smoothie with frozen berries, beet juice, and collagen protein powder.

Dinner: Vegetable soup (blended), with bone broth added. Drink stinging nettle tea.

Detoxing your Home

When I discuss cleansing your home, your mind, and your body, I make a very important point that you shouldn't be doing it all at once. When you are new to "cleaner or greener" living you can get overwhelmed. The key here is to go through every step at a comfortable pace. It's also important that you always have affordable options when you replace toxic products in your home. There are ways to make homemade non-toxic cleaning products, beauty products and personal products. For those, like myself, who want to make their lives easier there are plenty of green and clean products in health stores and online. The number of cleaning products being sold on the market now have grown exponentially as compared to when I started green-cleaning my home.

Just make sure it's not a brand that has an "Eco Friendly" label while not being human friendly.

Now, it's so delightful to go into stores or shop online and see so many products that are GMO-free, paraben-free, SLS-free, etc. We have come a long way.

It took me years, probably a decade, to detox my house, starting with the food products, to the cleaning products, to the beauty products, to the personal products, to the toothpaste, to the bedsheets, to the mattresses, to the water filters, to the air filters, etc. I'm still learning and loving it! Please, remember to detox your life slowly, but do start. It's like brushing your teeth. You know what happens if you don't!

It's becoming more popular to jump on the detox bandwagon. And why not? It's a wonderful idea. Since we are exposed to different toxins in our food, water, air, and anything that meets our skin we realize we need to cleanse. With all that pollution, it's no wonder why we are so toxic. A lot of chemicals, heavy metals, and parasites that enter our body remain hidden in different areas to cause all sorts of diseases and allergies. We don't even realize this until we are diagnosed with an illness. And, even at that point, many health care practitioners won't be able to find the root cause of your problem.

Detoxification helps clear toxins out of your body and it decreases the load of toxicity that your body is exposed to. This produces great health benefits, ranging from feeling well and having lots of energy to having great looking and healthy hair. A good detox program can help you clean and reset your system to bring about a happier, healthier, and more energetic you.

There are a lot of different cleanses and flushes on the market that promise to give you a clean bill of health. Just keep in mind that detoxification is not as simple as taking some type of herbal preparation. A good quality detox program is one that is safe, effective, and individually catered, just for you.

It's important to get your body prepared for a detox program. Once you start drawing out all the toxins from their hiding places, they then must exit from your body, otherwise you will feel very sick. If detoxing is making you sick, it may be that your excretory pathways are compromised and overwhelmed by such a large concentration of these toxins or those pathways weren't functioning at their optimal level to begin with; hence your situation.

Your first order of business is to correct the root causes. Those can include adrenal issues, gastrointestinal issues, chemical exposures, emotional issues, and others. And really, if you're going to put all that effort into improving your health, it only makes sense to do it right the first time.

Case Study:

A 37-year-old female with a high-stress job who had severe stomach cramps, infertility, and chronic nasal congestion came into our functional medicine practice. She started a functional medicine program and stopped after a few weeks because she didn't want to stop drinking caffeine and didn't want to start a gluten-free diet. After a few months she came back to restart the program. She was completely ready and very compliant. The detox program was done only after a successful adrenal and gut support. Slowly all the gut symptoms were disappearing. Nasal congestion stopped. She got pregnant one year later.

Although it's possible to do the program on your own, it's that much more helpful to have someone guide you through the entire process. A functional medicine expert is the perfect someone to create a detox program, since a big part of functional medicine is helping your body get back to balance and good health.

Basic and General Nutraceutical Protocol for Detox Support:

Do not try new supplements without discussing them with your physician or healthcare practitioner first.

- N-Acetyl-L-Cysteine 1 capsule after each meal
- Liver Support Phase one and two (ex, Amino Detox (DFH) 2 capsules three times daily and LV/GB(DFH) 1 capsule three times daily or HepatoDetox (Moss Nutrition) 1 capsule two to three times daily)
- Complete Mineral Support 1 capsule twice daily

Mold at Home

As I was learning about mold, I found out that mold is present in most homes, but they may be at levels that are considered acceptable. Some places have dangerous, toxic mold, making you exhausted, giving you brain fog, breathing issues, insomnia, bags under your eyes, and more. Constant attack by toxic mold can eventually lead to cases of asthma, thyroid disease, allergies, and autoimmune conditions.

If you have severe health problems due to mold exposure your doctor may start you on Cholestyramine and antifungal medication like fluconazole or itraconazole.

Basic and General Nutraceutical Protocol for Mold:

Do not try new supplements without discussing them with your physician or healthcare practitioner first.

- Oil of Oregano 1-2 capsules three times daily, depending on tolerability for two months
- S. Boulardii (ex, Floramyces by DFH or S.Boulardii by Garden of Life Original Medicine Line) 2 capsules three times daily for two months

- Acacia Gum and Activated Charcoal can be used for the short-term as binders

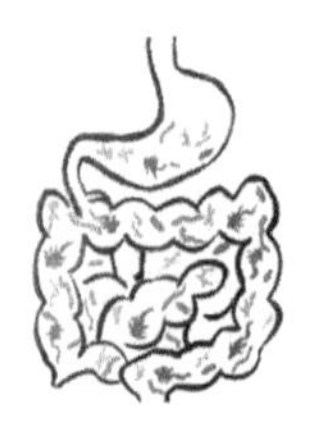

Chapter 11
MINDFULNESS IN IBDS

"Peaceful mind and peaceful digestion are your birthright."
– **Inna Lukyanovsky**

Don't like meditation? There are other options.

If you are not the biggest believer in mind-body connection, I'm not urging you to become one. I often get questions associated with mind-body and how I can be a pharmacist and still believe in it. Science already backs up many benefits of positive emotions, affirmation, and pre-conditioning. Also, science even backs up the benefits of energy fields with positive intention. Science will get more involved as we evolve into mindful modern-aged people. My suggestion to you is that if you don't believe it, you don't have to, but try the methods anyway. First, you have nothing to lose by trying—no side effects, that's for sure. Secondly, without any expectations, you may get a better result than someone who is going for it and expecting magic to happen.

The Power of Intentions

Did you know that the word "intention" has another meaning? It also means the healing process of a wound? In your case, that wound could be in your gut. Let's heal that gut.

Intentions can become the engine that drives your visions and goals. Intentions planted properly, like good seeds in organic soil, will yield healthy and clean fruit. And that fruit can be your healthy, beautiful tummy.

Think of an intention like the first sentence of your dream. What is it that you wish for? What would you like for your birthday on a health care scale? Start with that sentence and try making it in the least amount of words possible.

Setting an intention is like drawing up a business plan. You have your goals and then you go backwards trying to figure out the steps needed to accomplish your goals. You may not consciously figure it out, but your subconscious may take care of that for you. If you decide to heal, and your intention is strong, the required steps will follow.

Also, you must understand that the intentions should be created with a fun and light heart. If you feel heavy and negative, postpone setting your intention at a better time. But do seek the moment when you feel slightly more upbeat and ready to set your wonderful intentions.

These are samples of 10 gut-healing intentions for you to consider. Try these or make up your own and practice setting them each morning:

- Today, I intend to have great digestion.
- Today, I intend to think of myself first.
- Today, I intend to notice only good things around me.
- Today, I intend to have a smooth elimination of toxins.

- Today, I intend to absorb my nutrients properly.
- Today, I intend to dedicate time to eating without interruptions.
- Today, I intend to have a smooth bowel movement.
- Today, I intend to love my gut unconditionally.
- Today, I intend to make more time for me and rest as part of my lifestyle.
- Today, I intend to share my positive experiences.

Add more if you have something on your mind. Stay with it for a few moments longer to enhance that positive energy flow. And go on with your day noticing how much smoother your day turns out. Intention is stronger when it comes from a place of balance than if it arises from a sense of lack or need.

Important things about intentions:

1. Use positive words like calm, smooth, and peaceful. Try to stay away from words like "pain" unless you absolutely cannot find a substitute. For example, instead of using phrases like "pain-free" or "painless day" which still have the word "pain" in the phrase, substitute it for "smooth," "happy," or "calm tummy." The words themselves have energy that carries over into physical pain.
2. Try intention for short-term goals and plans. Thinking too far ahead can take away from immediate results and can get you out of sync. For example, the sample I use has the words, "Today, I intend," so it's specific for short term. If you start thinking in the future or start using the words, "in the future," you are taking away from the moment. The future isn't ever here. All we have is today.
3. When you intend for the same thing over and over, your mind may start wandering because you are now too familiar with this mind game. It's time to change things up. Write down new

intentions or rewrite your intentions in a different way but stay with the same point.

If you like to meditate, the perfect time to meditate is before or after you do your intending. Meditations don't need to be complicated. Just a few minutes of inhaling and exhaling, keeping your attention on the breath, will do it. The key here is to release the intentions while meditating to avoid any kind of thinking process going on in your head. Also, it's important to detach yourself from the outcome no matter what. Because if you don't, it can lead to destruction or disappointment. And there's no reason for it.

Emotional Freedom Technique (EFT) is used for IBDs.

I'm personally a big believer in EFT, since it works for me. I've recommended it to almost all of my clients, and it has worked for them as well. What's so special about EFTs and why are they something to consider adding to my recommendations and my program?

Emotional Freedom Technique, or tapping, is a self-help technique that involves tapping near the points where meridians of energy are located. These points are located around the body, followed in a certain sequence. EFTs are used to ease up anxiety and tension, resolve deep issues, help manage stress, decrease tension headaches, improve sleep, increase energy, reduce muscle and joint pain, improve focus and coordination, improve self-esteem and anxiety, improve mindfulness, and so much more. Tapping has been researched and studied by great investigators and the results are published in peer-reviewed journals.

The tapping technique was originally introduced in the 1980s–1990s as TFT (thought field therapy) by therapists who were so confident this method worked that they were able to successfully bring it out into the alternative medicine world. Their beliefs were that all thoughts and emotions are energy and the energy, whether it's positive or negative, will eventually manifest itself and affect the body.

I often see clients overwhelmed by fear, anxiety, and anger, and all those emotions prevent them from making steps toward healing. EFTs often release or ease the fear, and the clients often get empowered to go ahead with the healing program, recommendations, and nutritional changes.

Due to past traumas or overload of current illness, your body simply has less energy to trust, digest, and to process energies coming in, and those also include foods. EFT helps you clear those up.

How does EFT work? EFT focuses on energy flow that runs throughout the body. The flow of energy or meridians are used for tapping and yield powerful results. The method combines tapping of energy meridians with certain affirmations, almost like combining an Eastern medicine approach with Western psychotherapy.

What's the best way to perform EFT:

The following are basic steps used:

1. *Identifying the Issue*—In the case of IBD, name the emotions or the location of the pain. The goal is to focus on only one issue at a time for the most effects.
2. *Creating a Reminder Phrase*—For IBD patients, it could be something like a memory you had or a phrase you used before the symptoms started.
3. *Number on a Scale*—If you had to give a number from 0 to 10, what would it be for your physical or emotional pain? Re-evaluate after each round.
4. *Making a Clear Affirmation*—Make up an affirmation that helps you feel strong and pain-free. For example, "Even though I feel this pain in my gut [or your phrase], I deeply and completely

accept myself." While you repeat this statement, you start by tapping on your hand, specifically on the fleshy part on the outer side of your palm under the pinky finger (karate chop area).

5. *Tapping Sequence*—There are eight meridian points to be used in tapping. Using two fingers is best, usually the index and the middle finger, and apply constant taps. You'll need to speak out loud to stay focused and effective. The points to tap are in this order: top of the eyebrows, side of the eyes, under the eyes, under the nose, under the chin, under the collarbone, under the arm (for women it's where the bra strap is) and top of the head.
6. *Test the Scale Again*—Be honest with yourself and give a number on the scale of 0 to 10 on how you are feeling about that emotion or pain.
7. *Repeat if Necessary*—If you feel that you need to repeat because the scale didn't move, or it just moved slightly for you, go ahead and repeat.

Example of EFT recommended for Crohn's and colitis patients:

Karate Chop: Even though my tummy has pain and is reacting to so many foods, I'm grateful for this because it's showing me a signal. I will let my tummy know that I'm listening now, and I'm going to help my tummy rather than fight my body.

Even though my gut is so distressed, I send it soothing energy and love. I'm tapping to soothe this process and allow my body to heal.

Even though some foods don't agree with me right now, and my food list is so limited, I'm grateful for a strong body and I'm ready to heal my beautiful gut.

Top of the Head: Sorry tummy.

Eyebrow: Those foods are not easy to digest.

Side of the Eye: We have many solutions now.

Under the Eye: I'm getting balanced as you are receiving gut healing.

Under the Nose: And love, positive communications, and understanding

Chin: Tapping is like soothing support.

Collarbone: For the tummy and the soul.

Under the Arm: You don't have to do it all alone anymore.

Top of the Head: It was a lot to process.

Eyebrow: No wonder you didn't have a lot of energy to digest food.

Side of the Eye: I'm here with you now.

Under the Eye: We're clearing things as we tap.

Under the Nose: It's improving already.

Chin: And I'm so grateful to you.

Collarbone: I'm sure it's exhausting…

Under the Arm: But it's improving as we tap.

Top of the Head: I took a lot of emotions in.

Eyebrow: I wasn't sure how to deal with my emotions.

Side of the Eye: But I'm resolving it now.

Under the Eye: I'm going to improve.

Under the Nose: The tension is released.

Chin: I'm digesting foods better now.

Collarbone: I'll be thinking ahead about what foods would be good for us.

Under the Arm: So grateful for you, my tummy.

Top of the Head: Thank you for being so nurturing.

Hypnotherapy for IBDs

With a brain-gut regulation problem, your brain is so sensitive that it even over reacts to things that are normal in your body. Since you have been used to GI pain and discomfort for so long, the signals between the gut and the brain can get misinterpreted and result in more stress.

Hypnosis can effectively interfere with that dysregulation and be an effective addition to a functional medicine program for GI healing.

Hypnosis has been studied for IBDs, IBS, GERD, and many other gut problems. Hypnosis is no longer the process of mesmerizing clients into an unconscious state. It's so much more.

Brain-gut hypnotherapy is very directed and effective. A qualified hypnotherapist is able to reset your thinking patterns and help you refocus from the problem and pain to GI comfort and warmth. Most hypnotherapists or hypnotists will use cognitive behavioral therapy where *you* focus more on coping which impacts gut symptoms.

Mindfulness-based interventions have been studied as part of a healing method for inflammatory bowel disease. There have been eight significant articles written on hypnotherapy for IBD. The strongest effects of the mindfulness-based interventions were seen in overall quality of life and in anxiety/depression. So now, no one can really say that mind-body therapy doesn't work. There was some supporting data even with other psychosocial areas like physiological function and perceived stress. It's such an important supplemental treatment option for Crohn's and colitis patients.

Yoga for Crohn's/Colitis

Yoga is a great exercise for everyone. Yoga is especially great for patients with Crohn's disease, colitis and IBS. Some natural practitioners use yoga for pain reduction. My yoga instructor, Harini, is great. Her voice and attitude is very soothing and it feels as though the healing is starting before you even begin exercising. There are some studies suggesting that yoga can be beneficial for gastrointestinal disorders.

These are the yoga poses she suggested for IBDs/Crohn's disease patients:

Cobra position

- You need to lie on your stomach on the floor with your legs straight and your palms flat on the floor level with your chest.
- Breathe in and, as you breathe out, try to tighten your stomach and buttock muscles and slowly raise your chest and middle torso by pressing your palms and hips into the floor.
- Try to lift as far as you can without causing back pain, but the more flexible you are, the more you will be able to straighten your arms and raise your torso into full cobra.
- Hold for a few breaths then slowly roll back down to the start position.

Standing Forward Bend

This posture is supposed to help with digestion. Most Crohn's disease patients have digestion problems. This pose can stimulate the liver and kidneys. Standing forward bend can help relieve anxiety and mild depression.

- Start by standing up straight then, as you breathe out, slowly hinge forward at your hips.
- Then bend over with a straight back, stretching your spine out and away from your hips as you fold forward. If you're flexible enough, place your palms flat on the floor with your legs straight. If not, try bending your arms and hold onto your elbows and relax deeper into the stretch with each exhalation. Try staying in this posture for at least 30 seconds, breathing deeply throughout.

Spinal Twist

- Sit on the floor with your legs straight out in front of you and your hands on the floor behind your hips.

- Bend your right leg and place the foot flat on the floor on the outside of your left leg, just above knee height.
- If you can, bend your left knee so that the foot is resting near your right buttock; if not keep your left leg straight.
- Lift your left hand off the floor and cross it over your body, resting the elbow on the outside of your right knee and grasping your right ankle with your left hand. In this position, slowly twist your torso as far around to the right as you can while keeping your back straight and both sit bones on the floor. Your right hand should remain planted on the floor behind your right hip.
- Twist a little more with each exhalation and after at least three breaths, slowly unwind and repeat on the other side.

My journey with Crohn's disease started many years ago and it turned out to be a successful healing story. I tried many different options with the goal to heal. I knew that I would be healthy again, but that simply couldn't have been done without relaxation techniques.

Choose a relaxation technique that works for you. It must be something that you look forward to doing. If you want to switch things up later, that's perfectly fine. When you look forward to your relaxation technique, chances are your healing response will be that much better.

I would advise anyone, whose intention it is to heal, to continue and incorporate whatever technique you trust to help ground you. It could be praying, mediating, or breathing techniques. Being consistent with it will pay off.

One of the things that we often see is someone who's going from one practitioner to another, from one healer to the next, and getting no result. Those patients are so eager to heal, and they don't understand why nothing is working. This is very common because their point of concentration is on "nothing works" instead of "my goal is to heal, and I don't want to hear anything else." Come up with a positive goal and get with it.

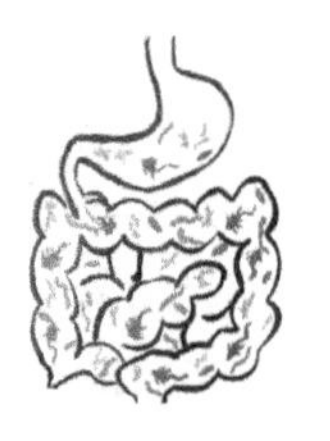

Chapter 12
I'M SCARED

"Fear is only as deep as the mind allows."
– Japanese Proverb

There Are So Many Obstacles to Change

When you learn that someone healed their Crohn's or colitis you get excited and even ready to try whatever they tried. You may even be ready to spend any kind of money for their healing secret, to eat whatever is necessary to heal and to do whatever it takes, except you fail to do it. It's hard to stick to a strict diet. It's hard to complete all the recommended steps, especially if you must give up the things that you enjoy. For example, your morning coffee, your late show, your staying up late habits, etc.

Giving up things that you love is hard. It's easier to just give up. I have my moments when I have to have that chocolate, or it's a happy occasion and that red wine looks so good. It's hard to be perfect all the time, yet it's possible to be good most of the time. Slipping up doesn't mean the end of the world, you get up the next day and make the next day your day to do your best. And often just giving up means giving up on your health. Your motivation can be your own kids, someone you love, someone to live for, etc.

I visit certain IBD groups and often see posts like this one:

"I visited a nutritionist and he suggested I get off dairy since he believes it aggravates my condition. But I only have cheddar, which is low on lactose, and yogurts, which provide you with probiotics. It's no big deal, right?" A bunch of people from the group replied to him that it's not a big deal, they eat dairy all the time. Some said not to listen to the nutritionist, others replied to change to lactose-free dairy, and I saw one reply out of dozens telling him to stop the dairy.

After reading all the replies, I could just see how satisfied the original poster would get. He didn't want to give up the food he enjoyed, he searched for a way to find an excuse not to give up dairy, and now he had found the validation not to. Our behavioral patterns are hard to break and breaking those will require discipline, work, and often guidance. Sometimes the guidance can be found through a group of like-minded people, the ones that are ready to do whatever it takes to heal their tummy. But often you get trapped in groups that look for excuses and would rather hide inside their disease—like this support group.

Just think about it, the guy visited a health care professional who specializes in this condition and highly recommended that the patient get off dairy. Why get home and look for support to continue your inflammatory eating habit rather than decide to follow advice?

When I get my clients who have been around the block and ask what diets they have tried, they may reply that nothing worked for them.

Not gluten-free, not dairy-free, not paleo. And when I ask how long they spent on those diets, their reply would be: "Oh, like an entire two weeks." Often we need to break those self-sabotaging behaviors to heal. Once you establish this self-control and self-help energy within yourself, you get great results.

Finding a great doctor may be hard enough. Finding a great doctor who resonates with your ideas on healing can be even harder, but it's not impossible. It will require some inquiring and at least a few appointments, but it is possible. You will know right away when the doctor isn't for you. It's almost like a dating game. If the chemistry isn't there, why bother? Your doctor should remain the alpha to make health care decision for your body, yet the doctor cannot be scaring you so much that you get a flare from the stress of the appointment. Your doctor appointment should not be a stressful event. Think of it as a tune-up appointment. Your body needs some fine-tuning and the doctor will make some recommendations. It's your right to politely ask for all possible alternatives and complementary options that the doctor believes have sufficient data to try. It's your right to ask your doctor if they are familiar with complementary options.

Take charge. You are the center of your own healing. Everything and everyone else is around *you*.

Your health is important to you and your loved ones. There's no one else on this planet, but you, that knows how you feel inside, both physically and emotionally. Learning to trust yourself and the process is an important step in healing. Whatever you decide to do will get you on a better path to heal.

It's crucial to make a great healing circle for yourself. You are the one in the center of the circle and you are the one who wants the results. The people around you, in that circle, are the health care practitioners (traditional and alternative), massage therapists, chiropractors, acupuncturists, detox specialists, and more. Your circle can contain just a few people or many. That would be entirely up to you. Make that circle comfortable. Fill the circle up with experienced, trained and reliable practitioners. Check their education and training and use your intuition to feel if they work for you or not. If the doctor doesn't seem to understand your health goals or is intimidating to you, then this may not be the doctor for you, even if it's a doctor with the best education from the most prestigious school in the country.

It's a good idea to have an upfront discussion with your doctor to find out if they believe in not just traditional, but also complementary options as well. If your doctor is not comfortable with that, then it's something you need to know. I sometimes discuss the medication and supplement list with my clients and often they give me a list of supplements that they didn't present to their doctor. Some clients are simply afraid that the doctor will "yell at them." That is completely unacceptable since some medications will interact with supplements. Some supplements will need to be taken a few hours apart from foods and medications. You'll need to create your health circle to comfortably include the entire list of foods, medications, supplements, herbs, and more, so a professional can check for interactions and go over them with you.

I sometimes have clients who do what's called "doctor hopping." That is another obstacle to healing. Most of these clients have psychological attachment issues with their disease. Once a client feels better or even much better, some of them become uncomfortable with themselves. Since they associated themselves with having the disease for so long, it became very strange to stop feeling ill. It became strange to feel better, to feel more energy, to have a healthy appetite, to have solid stools or to have no pain. They are not familiar with that territory and they are out of their comfort zone. For some clients it's a great transition but for others it's a scary one, to the point that they are ready to return to feeling comfortable again, even if it was physically painful. This may sound insane to you. How can someone that got better decide to turn back? And for those who are reading this book and already tried methods that sort of worked, you may not even realize that you've quit them because it felt uncomfortable on a subconscious level. It's not your fault. Our minds have a funny way of controlling many things. You may not understand why you are eating a third or fourth candy when you know you shouldn't have any at all. You may not understand why you are grabbing another cocktail when you shouldn't. Just the same way, you may not understand why you are going from practitioner to practitioner without getting results. But, the results are within you. Give one program a real chance, do whatever it is you have to do, do whatever is recommended, stay there until it works. This can become life changing.

I don't want to try another method because I don't want to feel disappointed

I am scared to start another program because it's too expensive

I am reluctant to start something to heal my gut because it's hard work

I am so uncomfortable to start anything new right now because it may not work

I am feeling so numb inside that I may not get the courage to start

I can no longer heal; I've tried everything

If any of this sounds familiar to you, I recommend appreciating all these emotions. Get the most strength from them. Remember how you feel, and draw up from these emotions to get to your next step. It should be a baby step, for sure. That's the only way to succeed here. You know how you can feel on the other side. How amazing it feels to be pain-free. How amazing it feels to get out of the house without looking for a bathroom on every corner. How amazing it feels to spend time with your kids, being all in. How amazing it is to have energy again? And boy, how I want this for you. For me it was a long process and I'd love this to be a much shorter journey for you by avoiding the mistakes I made and skipping some of those awful and scary social media recommendations. My book is here to bring you clarity, strength, and tools to heal your tummy.

All those doubts will start fading away as you go step-by-step from the first recommendation to the next, in that order. You'll transform into a person who can control many aspects of your health and maybe you'll become an amazing health advocate to others.

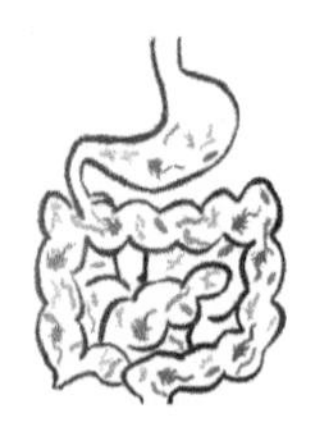

Chapter 13
THE HEALTHIEST YOU'VE BEEN

"All disease starts in the gut."
– **Hippocrates**

Program Tested Over and Over

It took many years, a lot of experience, excitement and drive to create my IBD-Free Program. I believe I'm following my mission by sharing my knowledge and guidance.

I—I am
I am in the center of my healing
B—Believe
Believe that you can heal

D—Decrease

Decrease or shut down the outside noise and overwhelming load of information

F—Find

Find the root cause

R—Reduce

Reduce the exposure to toxins, chemicals, heavy metals, and toxic thoughts

E—Eliminate

Eliminate pathogens, parasites, bacterial overgrowth, SIBO, and toxic foods

E—Empower

Empower yourself and equip your gut's microbiome with good bacteria, healing foods, appropriate nutraceuticals, and healing human connections to finally heal

The program I created for my IBD clients has this structure and it's recommended to be followed in a step-by-step process, because each next step depends on the one before it to be completed to work. The practical steps, recommendations, and protocols are within the IBD-FREE program. Individual recommendations can also be followed from the first step to the last:

I—I am

I am in the center of my healing. I can stay centered and refuse to be influenced by other people's criticism or doubts. My powerful subconscious knows that everything is all right and will be all right, even without knowing the details or timing of what will happen.

B—Believe

Believe that you can heal. Start believing it without doubts, questions, etc. Even if you don't believe that you can heal, repeat to yourself "I can heal," over and over, in the morning, during the day and before going to sleep. Write it down for yourself if necessary.

D—Decrease

Decrease or shut down the outside noise and overwhelming load of information. So many sites, groups, and forums share information that isn't credible. It's especially noticeable for me as a pharmacist, being able to interpret quickly whether an article, study, research, or paper has quality information. So, if you lack the scientific statistical knowledge base, consider finding one good reliable source and staying with that source.

F—Find

Find the possible root causes of your IBD—and those could be numerous. Those root causes can vary from adrenal problems, to blood sugar instability, to gut infections, to microbiome problems, to toxicity problems, and many more. A trained functional medicine practitioner should be able to dig through all of those.

R—Reduce

Reduce exposure to toxins, chemicals, heavy metals, and toxic thoughts. And that means learning more about your home, your area, your gut microbiome, and toxins in your gut. And don't forget to address toxic thoughts. They can play a detrimental role as well.

E—Eliminate

Eliminate pathogens, parasites, bacterial overgrowth, SIBO, and toxic foods. This alone can be a long process but as much as it's lengthy, that's how much this process will be rewarding. One client got rid of a common infection of H. Pylori and most of her IBD symptoms were eliminated.

E—Empower

Empower yourself and equip your gut's microbiome with good bacteria, healing foods, appropriate nutraceuticals, and healing human connections to finally heal. This is the most fun process because here you get to "play" with some good bacteria in your gut, feeding it the right kind of foods, sending it appropriate probiotics and making sure the pH of the body is perfectly alkaline. Natural supplements help a great deal, but they don't stand a chance if your participation isn't there. Nutraceuticals will help to a degree if you just want "another pill" to help you. But without getting involved in your gut healing, the supplements will have their limits.

As I was writing my first blog post on my journey with Crohn's disease website, I was thinking how exciting it would be to share all this knowledge and experience with fellow Crohn's and colitis patients. But something was always stopping me from writing the book. I thought, *Let me learn just a little bit more about IBD.* I thought that when I got my doctoral degree I'd be an authority to write the book. I thought, *let me just help more IBD clients and get even more experience,* and you know what? It took this long to finally write my book. And looking back, I should have written a book at every step of the way, and kept on writing more and more. You can never know everything. You can never please everyone. You can never get all the doctoral degrees and certifications possible. But I could have shared with my readers that they were not alone. I could have made a difference for someone long ago. So now with my doctorate in Pharmacy, almost a decade of experience with functional medicine, and with an experience as a Crohn's patient, I am finally there.

My book is my journey, which I know can help you set a good structure to start your healing. And while it's possible to do it alone with the information and the steps I'm giving you, it's great to have a guide. I know I wish I'd had that when I was diagnosed. All those unnecessary trials and errors could have been avoided.

One of my favorite phrases that my functional medicine mentor said was, "As functional medicine practitioners we can't prevent our clients from getting stressed. Stress is everywhere. Stress is the new 'norm.' But sure, we should be able to make sure stress doesn't get them sick or sicker." I am so happy to be able to do what I love doing in my practice. I review my client's cases, spending as much time as necessary, and my practice setting allows me to do that.

When you have guidance, you can become the healer for yourself and your family without having to experiment, but rather be equipped tips and a structural approach to healing. You can involve your entire family in the process of healing and the effect of that will be healthier kids and a healthier spouse. This can certainly be beneficial for everyone you love and care for. Once you start detoxing your body and your home, your loved ones will also benefit tremendously. Win-win situation.

Humans were made for communication. We thrive around people, and we get sick when very lonely. Once you get help and start feeling better, you naturally want to start sharing with other IBD patients, with your friends, your colleagues, etc. It will feel amazing to share your own healing story.

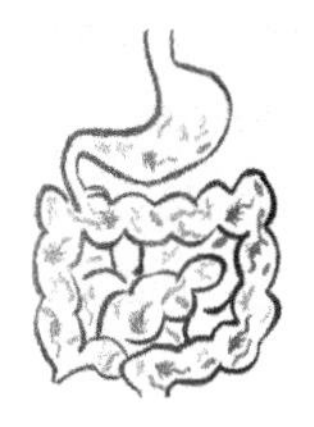

Chapter 14
USE TRUSTED RESOURCES

"There could never be enough good resources."
– Inna Lukyanovsky

Learning as We Go

If you want to start your own functional medicine healing, consider getting tested by reputable companies. Functional diagnostic companies have the research available on their websites, journals, articles, etc. The following are the companies I recommend using:

For Testing:

1. *Adrenal/Hormone Testing*
    - BioHealth Laboratory 800-570-2000
    - Dutch Testing 503-687-2050

2. *PCR technology stool testing*
   - o GI-MAP by Diagnostic Solutions Lab 877-485-53365-5336
   - o GI Effects by Genova Diagnostics
3. *SIBO Breath Testing Resources:* UNITED STATES (Direct patient ordering of Lactulose kits without a prescription is available from Direct Labs and True Health Labs in the US)
   - o 3 Hour Test:
     - Aerodiagnostics 844-681-9449
     - Biohealth Laboratory 800-570-2000
     - Breath Trackers/Quin Tron 800-542-4448
     - Direct Labs 800-908-0000
     - Genova Diagnostics 800-522-4762 (lab offers 2 & 3 hour tests)
   - o 2:15 Hour Test:
     - Commonwealth Diagnostics International 888-258-5966
   - o 2 Hour Test:
     - Genova Diagnostics 800-522-4762 (lab offers 2 & 3 hour tests)
4. Micronutrient Testing
     - SpectraCell Laboratories 800-227-5227
5. PubMed.com for studies available on the topic
6. EWG.org an environmental working group
7. IFM.org Institute for Functional Medicine

REFERENCES

Battat R, Kopylov U, et al Association Between Ustekinumab Trough Concentrations and Clinical, Biomarker, and Endoscopic Outcomes in Patients with Crohn's Disease. Clin Gastroenterol Hepatol. 2017 Mar 29. pii: S1542-3565(17)30386-5.

Bibiloni R, Fedorak RN, Tannock GW, et al. VSL#3 probiotic-mixture induces remission in patients with active ulcerative colitis. Am J Gastroenterol 2005;100:1539-46

Bousvaros A, Guendalini S, Baldassano R N. et al A randomized, double blind trial of Lactobacillus GG versus placebo in addition to standard maintenance therapy for children with Crohn's disease. Inflamm Bowel Dis 200511833–839.

C Prantera. Probiotics for Crohn's disease: what have we learned? Gut. 2006 Jun; 55(6): 757–759.

Campieri M, Rizzello F, Venturi A. et al Combination of antibiotic and probiotic treatment is efficacious in prophylaxis of post-operative recurrence of Crohn's disease: a randomized controlled study vs mesalamine. Gastroenterology 2000118A781

Caprilli R, Gassull MA, Escher JC et al. European evidence based consensus on the diagnosis and management of Crohn's disease: special situations. Gut 2006; 55 (Suppl 1): i36–58.

Clinical Care Pathway. http://cpms.bbinfotech.com/clients/aga_web_tools/interactive_0000542.html. American Gastroenterological Association 2017

Egeberg A1, Weinstock LB2, Thyssen EP2, Rosacea and gastrointestinal disorders: a population-based cohort study. Br J Dermatol. 2017 Jan;176(1):100-106.

Elmer GW. Probiotics: "living drugs." Am J Health Syst Pharm 2001;581101-1109

Faubion W A, Sandborn W J. Probiotic therapy with E. Coli for ulcerative colitis: take the good with the bad, Gastroenterology 2000118630–631.

Fedorak RN, Feagan BG, Hotte N, et al. The probiotic VSL#3 has anti-inflammatory effects and could reduce endoscopic recurrence after surgery for Crohn's disease. Clin Gastroenterol Hepatol. 2015 May;13(5):928-35.

Garcia Vilela E, De Lourdes De Abreu Ferrari M, Oswaldo Da Gama Torres H, et al. Influence of Saccharomyces boulardii on the intestinal permeability of patients with Crohn's disease in remission. Scand J Gastroenterol. 2008;43(7):842-8.

Gary R. Lichtenstein, MD, Stephen B. Hanauer, MD, William J. Sandborn, MD, et al, Management of Crohn's Disease in Adults. Am J Gastroenterol advance online publication, 6 January 2009.

Gionchetti P, Rizzello F, Helwig U. et al Prohylaxis of pouchitis onset with probiotic therapy: a double blind, placebo controlled trial. Gastroenterology 20031241202–1209

Gionchetti P, Rizzello F, Venturi A, et al. Oral bacteriotherapy as maintenance treatment in patients with chronic pouchitis: a double-blind, placebo-controlled trial. Gastroenterology 2000;119:305-9

Goldin BR, Gorbach SL. Clinical indications for probiotics: an overview. Clin Infect Dis. 2008;46(suppl)

Gong D, Gong X, Wang L et al, Involvement of Reduced Microbial Diversity in Inflammatory Bowel Disease. Gastroenterol Res Pract. 2016;2016:6951091.

Gorbach S L. Probiotics and gastrointestinal health. Am J Gastroenterol 200095(suppl)S2–S4.

Gurudu S, Fiocchi C, and Katz JA. Inflammatory bowel disease. Best Pract Res Clin Gastroenterol 2002;16:77-90.

Guslandi M, Giollo P, Testoni PA. A pilot trial of Saccharomyces boulardii in ulcerative colitis. Eur J Gastroenterol Hepatol 2003;15:697-8.

Guslandi M, Mezzi G, Sorghi M. et al Saccharomyces boulardii in maintenance treatment of Crohn's disease. Dig Dis Sci 2000451462–1464.

Hilsden RJ, Scott CM, Verhoef MJ. Complementary medicine use by patients with inflammatory bowel disease. Am J Gastroenterol 1998;93:697-701

Hilsden RJ, Verhoef MJ, Best A, Pocobelli G. Complementary and alternative medicine use by Canadian patients with inflammatory bowel disease: results from a national survey. Am J Gastroenterol 2003;98:1563-8

Hollander D, Vadheim C, Brettholz E. et al Increased intestinal permeability in patients with Crohn's disease and their relatives. Ann Intern Med 1986105883–885.

Klaus J1, Spaniol U, Adler G, Mason RA, Small intestinal bacterial overgrowth mimicking acute flare as a pitfall in patients with Crohn's Disease. BMC Gastroenterol. 2009 Jul 30;9:61.

Kornbluth A, Sachar D et al, Ulcerative Colitis Practice Guidelines in Adults: American College of Gastroenterology, Practice Parameters Committee, ACG PRACTICE GUIDELINES 2010

Kump P1, Högenauer C. Any Future for Fecal Microbiota Transplantation as Treatment strategy for Inflammatory Bowel Diseases? Dig Dis. 2016;34 Suppl 1:74-81

Laffin M1,2, Madsen KL2,3. Fecal Microbial Transplantation in Inflammatory Bowel Disease: A Movement Too Big to Be Ignored. Clin Pharmacol Ther. 2017 Oct;102(4):588-590.

Macfarlane GT, Cummings JH. Probiotics and prebiotics: can regulating the activities of intestinal bacteria benefit health? BMJ 1999;318:999-1003.

Mathisen, Stephanie. "Inflammatory Bowel Disease." British Society for Immunology, www.immunology.org/public-information/bitesized-immunology/immune-dysfunction/inflammatory-bowel-disease

Miele E, Pascarella F, Giannetti E. et al. Effect of a probiotic preparation (VSL#3) on induction and maintenance of remission in children with ulcerative colitis. Am J Gastroenterol 2009;104:437-43

Mimura T, Rizzello F, Helwig U, et al. Once daily high dose probiotic therapy (VSL#3) for maintaining remission in recurrent or refractory pouchitis. Gut 2004;53:108-14.

Plein K, Hotz J. Therapeutic effects of Saccharomyces boulardii on mild residual symptoms in a stable phase of Crohn's disease with special respect to chronic diarrhea - a pilot study. Z Gastroenterol 1993;31:129-34

Prantera C, Scribano M L, Falasco G. et al Ineffectiveness of probiotics in preventing recurrence after curative resection for Crohn's disease: a randomised controlled trial with Lactobacillus GG. Gut 200251405–409

Prantera C, Scribano M L. Crohn's disease: the case for bacteria. Ital J Gastroenterol Hepatol 199931244–246.

Rana SV1, Sharma S2, Kaur J2, Relationship of cytokines, oxidative stress and GI motility with bacterial overgrowth in ulcerative colitis patients. J Crohns Colitis. 2014 Aug;8(8):859-65.

Reinisch W. Fecal Microbiota Transplantation in Inflammatory Bowel Disease. Dig Dis. 2017;35(1-2):123-126.

Rembacken B J, Snelling A M, Hawkey P M. et al Non-pathogenic Escherichia coli versus mesalazine for the treatment of ulcerative colitis: a randomised trial. Lancet 1999354635–639.

Ricci JE Júnior1, Chebli LA, Ribeiro TC, Small-Intestinal Bacterial Overgrowth is Associated With Concurrent Intestinal Inflammation But Not With Systemic Inflammation in Crohn's Disease Patients. J Clin Gastroenterol. 2017 Jan 27.

Riquelme A J, Calvo M A, Guzman A M. et al Saccharomyces cerevisiae fungemia after Saccharomyces boulardii treatment in immunocompromised patients. J Clin Gastroenterol 20033641–43

Rutgeerts P, Geboes K, Peeters M. et al Effect of faecal stream diversion on recurrence of Crohn's disease in the neoterminal ileum. Lancet 1991338771–774.

Salvatore S, Heuschkel R, Tomlin S, et al. A pilot study of N-acetyl glucosamine, a nutritional substrate for glycosaminoglycan synthesis, in paediatric chronic inflammatory bowel disease. Aliment Pharmacol Ther 2000;14:1567-79

Sartor R B. Enteric microflora in IBD: pathogens or commensals? Inflamm Bowel Dis 1997323–35.

Sartor R B. Role of intestinal microflora in initiation and perpetuation of inflammatory bowel disease. Can J Gastroenterol 19904271–277

Shafran I1, Burgunder P. Adjunctive antibiotic therapy with rifaximin may help reduce Crohn's disease activity. Dig Dis Sci. 2010 Apr;55(4):1079-84

Shanahan F. Probiotics and inflammatory bowel disease: is there a scientific rationale? Inflamm Bowel Dis20006107–115.

Snydman Dr. The safety of probiotics. Clin Infect Dis 2008;46(suppl)

Sokol H, Pigneur B, Watterlot L, et al. Faecalibacterium prausnitzii is an anti-inflammatory commensal bacterium identified by gut microbiota analysis of Crohn disease patients. Proc Natl Acad Sci U S A. 2008 Oct 28;105(43):16731-6.

Steed H, Macfarlane GT, Blackett KL, et al. Clinical trial: the microbiological and immunological effects of synbiotic consumption - a randomized double-blind placebo-controlled study in active Crohn's disease. Aliment Pharmacol Ther. 2010 Oct;32(7):872-83.

Stenson WF, Korzenik J. Inflammatory Bowel Disease. In: Yamada T, ed. Textbook of Gastroenterology. 4th ed. Philadelphia, PA: Lippincott Williams & Wilkins; 2003.

Tiao DK1, Chan W, Jeganathan J, Chan JT. Inflammatory Bowel Disease Pharmacist Adherence Counseling Improves Medication Adherence in Crohn's Disease and Ulcerative Colitis. Inflamm Bowel Dis. 2017 Aug;23(8):1257-1261.

Tursi A, Brandimarte G, Giorgetti GM, et al. Low-dose balsalazide plus a high-potency probiotic preparation is more effective than balsalazide alone or mesalazine in the treatment of acute mild-to-moderate ulcerative colitis. Med Sci Monit 2004;10:PI126-31

Venturi A, Gionchetti P, Rizzello F, et al. Impact on the composition of the faecal flora by a new probiotic preparation: preliminary data on maintenance treatment of patients with ulcerative colitis. Aliment Pharmacol Ther 1999;13:1103-8.

Wilson A, et al. Genetic predictor helps IBD patients avoid drug-induced pancreatitis Aliment Pharmacol Ther. 2017;doi:10.1111/apt.14483.January 11, 2018

ACKNOWLEDGMENTS

I would like to thank my incredible parents, my husband, and my boys. Thanks to my dad, who is at 70 years of age writing a math book with his own newly developed quick learning technique. Thanks to my mom who took care of it all while I was sick as a dog and is still going strong taking care of things when I'm all swallowed in my practice. Thanks to my husband who made me believe that I will be fine no matter what. Thanks to my boys who gave me the drive every day to continue my wonderful journey.

I am also very grateful for my amazing clients who taught me how to be a great listener, good healer, and a true servant at heart.

To the Morgan James Publishing team: Special thanks to David Hancock, CEO & Founder for believing in me and my message. To my Author Relations Manager, Margo Toulouse, thanks for making the process seamless and easy. Many more thanks to everyone else, but especially Jim Howard, Bethany Marshall, and Nickcole Watkins.

ABOUT THE AUTHOR

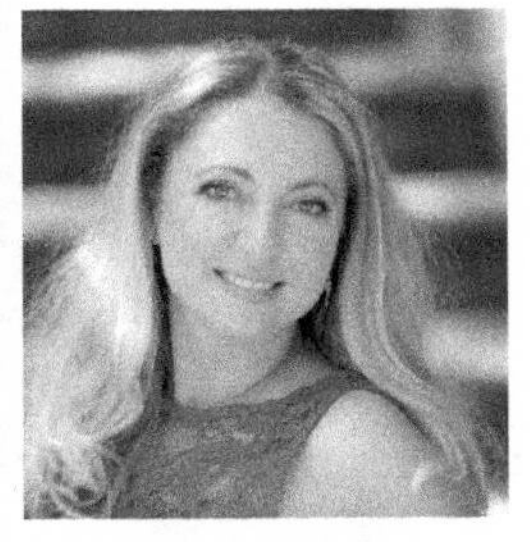

Inna Lukyanovsky is a Doctor of Pharmacy, an expert in complementary medicine options for gut health, and a Crohn's patient in full remission. Her career started as a traditional pharmacist and her mission later became to heal herself and help others with IBD.

During her time as a certified geriatric consultant pharmacist, Dr. Inna worked in a nursing home setting as part of an interdisciplinary team. She consulted on thousands of chronic, autoimmune, and other complicated cases which mainly incorporated pharmaceutical medications. After a short period of time, Dr. Inna was able to advise and influence the use of vitamin, mineral, and micronutrient supplementation for the nursing home residents. She became an expert in clinical pharmacology and familiar with identifying drug-related problems.

After fourteen years of researching Crohn's disease, colitis, and other digestive disorders, she is now combining the newest clinical information with her expertise and personal experience to launch a program to help digestive disease sufferers. Dr. Inna is also working on root cause and analysis-based protocols for her clients.

Since opening her practice, Real Health Solutions, she has helped hundreds of clients with their IBD, digestive problems, hormone imbalances, and other chronic conditions that could not have been resolved by traditional medicine alone. Dr. Inna successfully incorporates her extensive knowledge of functional medicine into every case that comes into her practice. She is truly passionate about helping people regain their health, vibrancy, and joy for life. She lives with her husband and three sons in Marlboro, New Jersey.

Website: realhealthsolutionsllc.com and DigestiveReset.com coming soon
Email: Inna@DigestiveReset.com
Facebook: https://www.facebook.com/realhealthsolutions/
Twitter: https://twitter.com/RealHealthSol
LinkedIn: https://www.linkedin.com/in/dr-inna-lukyanovsky-pharmd-4b204a67/
Instagram: https://www.instagram.com/innalukypharmd/

THANK YOU

Thanks for reading! I'd love to hear more about your gut healing stories, so please email me your comments at Inna@DigestiveReset.com.

I know that I'll always be learning, because my mission is to help, to teach, and to resolve your gut problems. And we are advancing to newer diagnostic tools, newer technology, newer genomic research, and newer microbiome research, even as you read this book. I am certainly planning to keep up with the research. This will prevent my brain from developing Alzheimer's, and it will make yours truly a reputable gut expert source.

A big thank you to you for trusting your gut and giving my book a chance. Healing your gut may just be a beginning to doing bigger and better things in your life. Healing your gut will mean more time with your kids. Healing your gut will mean being able to go out without looking for a bathroom. Healing your gut will mean being able to work more and be more productive. Healing your gut will mean more sexy time with your partner. Healing your gut will mean more energy for you! Healing your gut will mean getting the healthiest version of you!

My wish is for you to have all those things without the trial and errors, mistakes and disappointments. You deserve a healthy, strong, impermeable intestine.

FREE VIDEO CLASS: As a token of gratitude to thank you for reading, I would like to share a video class on gut healing with you.

You can find it here: http://www.realhealthsolutionsllc.com/digestive_reset/

FOR THE DEVELOPING WORLD
LIBRARY
FOR ALL
DIGITAL LIBRARY